B
METABOLIC
THERAPY
in the prevention and control of CANCER

a technical manual

Compiled by
PHILLIP DAY

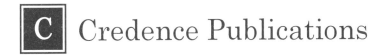

Credence Publications

TABLE OF CONTENTS

"I know of nothing so potent in producing ill-health as improperly constituted food. It may therefore be taken as a law of life, infringement of which shall surely bring its own penalties, that the single greatest factor in the acquisition of health <u>is perfectly constituted food</u>. Given the will, we have the power to build in every nation a people more fit, more vigorous and competent; a people with longer and more productive lives, and with more physical and mental stamina than the world has ever known." **Sir Robert McCarrison, Chairman of the Post-Graduate Medical Education Committee at Oxford University**

"We concentrate on consistency without much concern of what it is we are being consistent about, or whether we are consistently right or wrong. As a consequence, we have been learning a great deal about how to follow an incorrect course with the maximum of precision." **Deutscher, W, *Social Problems*, University of Manchester (UK) Institute of Science and Technology course hand-out**

INTRODUCTION
by Phillip Day
Credence Research

It is with great pleasure that I write to introduce the following research. However I do so with the marked poignancy that the chief pillars of the following information have been in the public domain in excess of fifty years and remain largely unheeded by our medical experts, many of whom are, as ever, fixated on the cure of cancer rather than its prevention. The aim of my organisation, Credence, is to report research that has failed to make its vital and *prominent* appearance either in the medical literature or through the mass communications media because of political or economic constraints, such as they are perceived. The purpose of this technical report is to encourage the re-education of the public and its physicians on cancer in all its forms, and thereby encourage and engender no more or less a goal than the total eradication of cancer in societies where this scourge is epidemic. To accomplish this with a high degree of success, three areas of education and action need to be urgently addressed: that of what cancer actually is, how to prevent it, and lastly, how to eradicate it in current patients, howsoever late-term in their illness.

The answers to many diseases previously fatal to mankind came through the age-old study of what worked and what didn't. This is the very nature and essence of science, or knowledge gained. Backroom boys fooling around in the lab, trying stuff out, blowing holes in the ceiling, learning from their successes and failures. Aye, as Shakespeare would remark, but here's the rub. History has shown a marked trend in human pride where, on more than one occasion, man has overlooked, fudged, prejudiced and, perhaps more significantly, *ignored* the obvious and unprofitable in favour of his often frenzied search for the answer within the technical and the brilliant, thereby increasing his own stature and income within his noble profession, and earning himself the approbation of his peers.

Leo Tolstoy astutely observed: *"I know that most men, including those at ease with problems of the greatest complexity, can seldom accept even the simplest and most obvious truth, if it would oblige them to admit the falsity of conclusions which they have delighted in explaining to colleagues, proudly taught to others, and which they have woven, thread by thread, into the fabric of their lives."*

Knowledge is a pride thing. Always has been.

For the first time, you are about to read a unique and comprehensive technical reference on a key series of nutritional treatments for cancer, complete with their total scientific justifications, which have been largely embargoed by traditional medicine in their search for the technical and complicated answers to cancer. This reference guide is not just for the benefit of physicians, practitioners and scientists, but also for members of the public, who have directly and indirectly helped to fund such ground-breaking work. The fact that this information has to come from a published source other than those provided by accepted medical journals, speaks volumes on just how *political* and *economic* an animal cancer has become. This reference book is designed to draw together the myriad research that has necessarily sprung out of mankind's honest desire to eliminate from its cultures a disease that has destroyed millions. The fact though that this information has been a matter of public knowledge for decades, and yet has not made it into general oncological practice, is perhaps one of the greatest scandals in medical and social history. The political and socio-economical reasons why this has happened, and continues to happen to this day, are discussed in some detail in my book *Cancer: Why We're Still Dying to Know the Truth.*

Scurvy, a disease that had slaughtered millions, was finally laid to rest only after science eventually accepted its nutritional causation. Science took many centuries to accomplish this paradigm shift in thinking, even after Jacques Cartier, Richard Hawkins and other explorers explained the simple nutritional prophylactic to their medical peers with all the understanding they could muster of their day. Yet the establishments heeded them not, and millions continued to die as a result.

Who were these millions? Were they not somebody's daughter, somebody's son? Has antiquity removed their laughter, their vibrancy and their love from us? Has history's effect hardened us to the lessons of the past by rendering the victims of history's mistakes an inscrutable sepia, the dust of their memory and echo of their passion for life blowing away with the sands of time? Are we still committing the mistakes of the past, having learned nothing from them to enhance our future?

Well known behavioral authority Anthony Robbins remarks: *"The past does not equal the future."* Robbins means that we hold in our hands today many keys that can change our world wonderfully and exponentially in so many ways. The question is, *will we choose to use those keys to unlock a new future*, or will we continue to suffer what we must suffer?

This book – this key - is of such strategic importance to the future of humanity that I spend ten months of every year away from my family and loved ones and travel the world educating people on how to use this key to prevent or survive a painful and unnecessary death. Contained within these following pages are the answers to a disease that has killed more people than have perished in all wars *ever*. To put this into perspective, imagine the breathtaking arrogance of a book that purported to contain the information that could end all war, and then imagine the significance of that book to humankind if the information contained within it were found to be true.

This book is all about an approach to cancer, its treatment and prevention, that continues to anger the medical, chemical and political establishments – which, if you think about it, is always a sign that science is on to something. Some say this approach is 'unique' and 'new', but I prefer to call it for what it is - a welcome return to the study of how humans used to exercise personal control over their own healthy destiny, before they were told by science they could not hope to survive without the 'new medical technology'.

Ironically, it is this same medical technology that has succeeded in some areas so spectacularly, while utterly and tragically failing in so many others. In my book *Health Wars*, I report research from around the world demonstrating that Western healthcare in many of the industrial societies has now reached the third leading cause of death. 225,000 Americans are routinely killed every year by Western healthcare, according to estimates published by the Journal of the American Medical Association (vol. 284, 26th July 2000). In Britain, the official figure of 40,000 per annum is far higher, if one examines the proper markers. In 1998, 1 in 5 Australians were reported killed by their healthcare system, through incorrect drug-prescribing, botched medical procedures, infections in hospitals and, the main killer, <u>correct</u> drug prescribing ('non-error, negative effects of drugs'). In the *Beijing Morning Post*, 28th September 2000, research shows that traceable iatrogenic deaths amount to 200,000 each year in that country (with many cases going unreported in the provinces). Also that 60-80% of China's 10 million deaf-mute cases have now been related to the use of inappropriate medicine.

Why is modern medicine failing so conspicuously with cancer and other degenerative diseases, and worse, discovering itself guilty of its own unique slaughter of the citizenry? One need look no further than the fact that doctors receive almost no formal training in nutrition. When one appreciates that degenerative diseases are metabolic and/or toxin-related in causation, which research is amply demonstrated in the scientific literature and summarised in *Health Wars*, one sees that doctors are simply not being trained to understand the underlying metabolic problems of the diseases they face, which can be treated effectively, even in their late stages, or completely prevented, using simple, and unfortunately un-patentable nutrition.

It is the aim of this manual to introduce the reader to the exciting nutritional concepts of cancer prevention and treatment. Also, the environmental poisonings that contribute so tragically to cancer need also to be made prominent here. Many medical scientists have come to trivialise the environmental chemical and radiological causes of cancer, notwithstanding the fact that their connection with many of the cancers is well established. It must also be pointed out that the very industry responsible for producing and selling chemicals, which routinely kill and maim the public, is the same industry that also manufactures the public's medicines. Can one expect the chemical and medical industries to gain a morality on this issue overnight, hamstrung as they are by stark conflicts of interest?

The urgent call for reform needed to prevent further tragedy on the scale we face must come from the public itself, in full support of those physicians who desire to be allowed to practise metabolic medicine[1] free of persecution and restrictive legislation, in addition to their use of mainstream existing modalities, which have demonstrated a clinical track-record of efficacy.

Medical science has known for years that the answers to heart disease, cancer, stroke and other illnesses lie completely in nutrition and lifestyle changes, not radical surgeries, toxic drugs or radiation. To prove this point, *Health Wars* highlights well-studied cultures alive today who do not suffer from these health problems, when kept in isolation from Western diets, Western medicine and Western lifestyle practices. Interestingly, we tend to call these peoples 'primitive' and 'less developed'. But they know enough to ensure that they survive in sterling health, in many cases to over 100 years of age, through making deliberate use of certain nutritional and environmental practices. The authorities know this too, yet have consistently ignored the vast body of eminently researched and published evidence indicating the benefits of pro-active nutrition, clean organic foods and water and a detoxified environment in the treatment and palliation of the public's many cancer sufferers.

A reform of the present ineffective and grossly finance-inflated health system is inevitable and currently underway. The public can do much to precipitate this process through becoming educated and politically active in even just the basic issues of nutrition and health. An effective healthcare industry must participate actively in this process and have nutrition at its heart. This is the most basic

---

[1] Metabolic medicine is sometimes referred to as 'Ortho-Molecular' medicine, after 'ortho' (correct), 'molecular' (molecules); or 'putting the correct molecules into the body so the body may heal and take care of itself'. This approach accepts and celebrates the fact that the body is a self-healing mechanism well capable of repairing and sustaining itself, if given the raw materials and the environment to do so.

body science. We are what we eat and absorb. Why would this science NOT be taught to doctors? Why indeed.

It is as if the monumental studies and conclusions which follow have been frozen in time, cryogenically suspended, as it were, by a medical establishment unwilling to accept the inevitable nutritional paradigm shift it has sought for decades to belittle and malign. And while such political considerations and analyses are not the main subject, nor intrinsic part of this work, the reader must bear uppermost in their mind the context in which such research was performed and reported, often in the harshest and most critical of professional conditions. Such research, of course, while decades old, remains in its observations, if not in its stentorian conclusions, as true today as it ever was. This single fact must never be overlooked.

The combined works of the scientists which follow, in addition to the countless reams of technical data on this same subject (for reasons of brevity and space not reported here), paint a forward-looking and extremely heartening picture of the future of cancer medicine – one in which the extreme pain of cut, slash and burn allopathics gives way to the healing, non-toxic and nutritional approaches, which will finally defeat and bury forever the old and implacable cancer adversary.

In a sense, the ultimate irony of cancer is that the research covered in the following chapters will have brought mankind back to his beginnings, where environments were once pristine, food organic, soils mineral-rich and properly constituted, and water the refreshing, uncontaminated renewer of the constant cycle of life. Dare we imagine, in the final analysis of the Rise and Fall of Cancer, that the most obdurate foe, the most stubborn and persistent enemy in the War on Cancer proved not to be the disease itself, in all its manifestations, but the reluctance of some of the most brilliant minds in science to take Tolstoy's courage and walk with wonder through the open door presented to them.

Today, we all have a chance to be great; to re-examine the motivations and desires that originally led us fresh-faced and all-conquering into the field of healing; to contemplate the legacy that each of us will leave behind, which will mark forever the achievements of our lifetime; to rise above the flawed and human nature of man, to offer real hope where before lay only death; to see if these things are so.

Will we?

ABOUT THIS AUTHOR

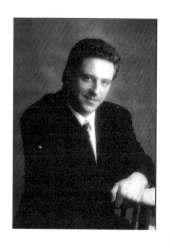

Phillip Day was born in England in 1960. He was educated at Selwyn and Charterhouse and throughout his '20s had a successful entrepreneurial career founding businesses in sales, advertising and marketing. With a firm grounding in business and the ways of the media, Phillip's research career began after he became interested irl human behaviour and wars going on in the realms of health and politics over issues that were being deliberately withheld or misreported to the public. His research into AIDS, cancer and other diseases, reporting the key work of scientists from all over the world, has spanned over a decade and a half and culminated in books and worldwide speaking tours that have captured the public's imagination. He is author, co-author or compiler of the following titles:

CANCER: WHY WE'RE STILL DYING TO KNOW THE TRUTH, HEALTH WARS
WORLD WITHOUT AIDS
FOOD FOR THOUGHT

Phillip heads up the publishing and research organisation Credence, which draws on the work provided by researchers from around the world. Credence's intention is to work with the establishments and organisations concerned to resolve these life-threatening issues, and to provide the necessary information for citizens to make their own informed choices in these vital matters. He is also Chief Executive of the Campaign for Truth in Medicine, a global organisation dedicated to precipitating much-needed reform into the health industry. Phillip Day currently lives in Kent, England.

METABOLIC THERAPY – AN OVERVIEW
Examining the Cancer Landscape
by Phillip Day

Cancer, the second leading killer in most Western industrialised nations, is a disease which has crept from an incidence rate of around 1 in 500 in 1900 to between 1 in 2 to 3 today. Over 600,000 people are expected to die from cancer in America in 2002, and yet, in spite of supposedly the brightest and the best walking the corridors of our leading cancer research institutions, armed with the latest technology and limitless budgets, the incidence rates for cancer continue to rise.

Breast cancer serves as a poignant yardstick. This type of malignancy is now the leading cause of death in women between the ages of 35 and 54. In 1971, a woman's lifetime risk of contracting breast cancer was 1 in 14.[2] Today it is 1 in 8. *Rachel's Environment and Health Weekly*, No. 571 reports: *"More American women have died of breast cancer in the past two decades than all the Americans killed in World War 1, World War 2, the Korean War and Vietnam War combined."*

The amazing thing is, most physicians in the world today have absolutely no idea what cancer is, or even how it is contracted. Some believe cancer is virus-related. Others believe the cause is parasites. Others yet examine the environmental causal link.

Let's look at what society generally knows about cancer and see how it stacks up with the truth. Most believe that:

- Cancer is a serious disease that kills those suffering from the life-threatening variants, such as lung, breast, bone, colorectal and liver.
- Cancer can only be treated with chemotherapy, radiation treatments and radical surgeries to poison or break up tumours, or physically remove them altogether.

---

[2] Epstein, Samuel S & David Steinman *The Breast Cancer Prevention Program*, Macmillan, USA, www.preventcancer.com

- These cancer treatments sometimes work and sometimes don't. No one can be sure who will survive and who won't.
- Cancer is caused by genetics, smoking, and other less well understood or known environmental causes.
- We still don't have the cure for cancer.
- The cancer charities and famous pop and TV stars are doing a superb job raising money to help with the drug research to combat and defeat cancer.
- Cancer appears to be a complex disturbance of cells in our bodies which mutate and then begin an uncontrollable proliferation. No one really knows what cancer is at the moment.

During the twelve years that I and my fellow researchers conducted our investigation into the cancer industry, what we found dispelled any illusions that cancer medicine was working in any way for the benefit of humanity. Here is what we found:

- The proof behind what cancer actually is and how to combat it effectively has been known for almost a century.
- Cancer is a healing process that hasn't terminated upon completion of its task.
- Cancer cells are pre-embryonic stem cells that have been stimulated by estrogen in our bodies to form trophoblast healing cells. It is these trophoblast cells that may progress to form 'cancer' cells if the trophoblastic multiplication of these cells (the healing process) is not halted.
- These rogue healing processes are started when our bodies become damaged in various ways. For instance, smoking damages the back of the throat and the lungs, resulting in site-specific healing processes that may or may not stop. Viruses, bacteria, mobile phones, physical blows, a toxic environment and chemical causations can all initiate healing processes in our bodies. In the event that a healing process is not terminated, healing trophoblast cells continue to proliferate to form a tumour.
- All cancers can be traced to ENVIRONMENTAL- OR LIFESTYLE-RELATED CAUSATIONS that damage our bodies, initiating a healing process that may not stop. We

can say 'ALL' because there are at least 18 different peoples on Earth today who do not suffer from cancer. Many of these cannot record even one victim of the disease in their entire culture. By this definition, cancer can be deemed preventable.

- The reasons why these peoples do not contract cancer are entirely known, yet this information, and the top researchers who discovered it, have been deliberately vilified by the mainstream science establishment.

- Orthodox medicine has waged an effective and relentless war against this life-saving knowledge to prevent its widespread dissemination and thus forestall an attack on the highly profitable cancer industry. There are more people today making a living out of cancer than are dying from it. The cancer industry turns over in excess of $200 billion annually.

- Cancer charities are fund-raising institutions for the pharmaceutical combines whose livelihoods depend on the continuance of cancer. Thus we see all efforts made to *wage* the war on cancer, not win it. In the event that cancer were vanquished, millions around the world would need to retrain. Cancer charities have no interest in knowing the truth about cancer - my organisation can vouch for that. Their job is to raise as much money as possible through the emotional showcasing of the heart-rending consequences of cancer, thereby stimulating the public to give more money.

- There is no evidence that chemotherapy and radiation treatments extend life in the major epithelial cancers, which are the majority of the cancers striking us today, *although these two treatments can and do sometimes effect a reduction in tumour size.* In a small minority of cases, as with some testicular and childhood cancers, efficacy with these treatments may be shown. Radiation and chemotherapy on the other hand have long been known to compromise the body's immune system, leading to the progressive degradation of the patient's health.

- Chemotherapy drugs are cytotoxic, meaning that they indiscriminately poison the cells in our body that multiply the most rapidly (cancer cells). However, certain immune system cells, such as our T and B lymphocytes, are also targeted, as these multiply rapidly too, contributing to our body's inability to fight opportunistic diseases that may come upon us as a result of the treatment.

- Radiations treatments harm the body, often leading to the production of more healing trophoblast. Radiation has been recognised to foster aggressive cell lines and in certain cases actually accelerate tumour growth.
- Cancer is a chronic, metabolic deficiency disease that is exacerbated by general mineral depletion in the food chain and the missing nitriloside dietary element. Cultures, whose diets are rich in essential nutrients and the nitrilosides, suffer no cancer in their peoples, provided they are living in toxin-free environments.

THE POLITICS OF BIG CANCER AND THE
FAILURE OF CONVENTIONAL TREATMENTS

Let's review some startling comments made by insiders to illustrate the point that the shameful corporate story surrounding cancer has long been known and written about by honest physicians who see major mischief afoot. Also included in this section is the compelling truth that conventional cancer treatments are not extending life in the major cancers striking us.

One such leading critic of the cancer industry has been Dr Samuel S Epstein, chairman of the Cancer Prevention Coalition and a world-renowned toxicologist and Professor of Occupational and Environmental Medicine at the University of Illinois Medical Center in Chicago. Epstein's relentless attacks against corporate vested interests in the chemical and medical industries concerning the avoidable causes of cancer have led to the public gaining a far wider knowledge of these issues. Epstein has no hesitation in indicting 'Cancer Inc.', comprising the American Medical Association, the National Cancer Institute, the American Cancer Society (ACS), the cancer charities and the pharmaceutical industry, as well as other cancer administrative bodies elsewhere in the world, for losing the winnable war against cancer. Epstein contends:

"We are not winning the war against cancer, we are losing the war. The number of Americans getting cancer each year has

escalated over recent decades, while our ability to treat and cure most common cancers has remained virtually unchanged.

The National Cancer Institute and the American Cancer Society have misled and confused the public and Congress by repeated false claims that we are winning the war against cancer – claims made to create public and Congressional support for massive increases in budgetary allocations."[3]

Quentin D Young, MD, president of the American Public Health Association, agrees with Epstein and highlights the chief environmental causes of cancer, which must be addressed if we are to turn the tide on the disease:

"Billions of public dollars are being misspent in an ill-conceived 'war on cancer' – a war we are losing because we are not addressing the increasingly carcinogenic environment that man has created. We have introduced these creations into our water and air, our food chain, our habitation, our workplace, and into the products produced there. In failing to allocate these resources for prevention, we are fighting the wrong war."[4]

John Cairns, professor of microbiology at Harvard University, recorded in his scathing 1985 critique in *Scientific American*: *"Aside from certain rare cancers, it is not possible to detect any sudden changes in the death rates for any of the major cancers that could be credited to chemotherapy.* <u>*Whether any of the common cancers can be cured by chemotherapy has yet to be established*</u>*."*

Making the point that chemotherapy is *not* curative, and actually has very little effect on the major cancers, Dr Martin F Shapiro stated in the *Los Angeles Times* that *"...while some oncologists inform their patients of the lack of evidence that treatments work... others may well be misled by scientific papers that express unwarranted optimism about chemotherapy. Still others respond*

---

[3] Epstein, Samuel *The Politics of Cancer Revisited*, East Ridge Press, USA 1998. www.preventcancer.com

[4] Epstein, Samuel, *The Politics....* Ibid.

to an economic incentive. <u>Physicians can earn much more money running active chemotherapy practices than they can providing solace and relief… to dying patients and their families</u>."[5]

Alan C Nixon, PhD, erstwhile president of the American Chemical Society, declares that *"…as a chemist trained to interpret data, it is incomprehensible to me that physicians can ignore the clear evidence that chemotherapy does much, much more harm than good."*

Oncologist Albert Braverman MD told the world in 1991 that *"…no disseminated neoplasm* (cancer) *incurable in 1975 is curable today… Many medical oncologists recommend chemotherapy for virtually any tumor, <u>with a hopefulness undiscouraged by almost invariable failure</u>."*

Christian Brothers, a retail organisation forcefully shut down by the American Food & Drug Administration (FDA) in 2000, states: *"In 1986, McGill Cancer Center scientists sent a questionnaire to 118 doctors who treated non-small-cell lung cancer. More than 3/4 of them recruited patients and carried out trials of toxic drugs for lung cancer. They were asked to imagine that they themselves had cancer, and were asked which of six current trials they themselves would choose. 64 of the 79 respondents would not consent to be in a trial containing cisplatin, a common chemotherapy drug. <u>Fifty-eight found all the trials unacceptable</u>. <u>Their reason</u>? <u>The ineffectiveness of chemotherapy and its unacceptable degree of toxicity</u>."* [6]

Dr Ralph Moss was the Assistant Director of Public Affairs at probably America's most famous cancer research institution, Memorial Sloan Kettering in Manhattan. He states: *"In the end, there is no proof that chemotherapy in the vast majority of cases actually extends life, and this is the GREAT LIE about*

---

[5] *Los Angeles Times*, 9th January 1991
[6] Christian Brothers, www.christianbrothers.com. Site now suspended by US Department of Justice action.

18

chemotherapy, *that somehow there is a correlation between shrinking a tumor and extending the life of a patient.*"[7]

Walter Last, writing in *The Ecologist*, reports: *"After analysing cancer survival statistics for several decades, Dr Hardin Jones, Professor at the University of California, concluded in 1975 that "...patients are as well, or better off untreated." Jones' disturbing assessment has never been refuted. What's more, three studies by other researchers have upheld his theory."*[8]

Professor Charles Mathe, French cancer specialist, makes this astonishing declaration: *"If I contracted cancer, I would never go to a standard cancer treatment centre. Cancer victims who live far from such centres have a chance."*[9]

From another angle, Dr John Gofman's mammoth research attacks 'preventative' measures, such as routine mammograms, for causing the very illness they are designed to prevent:

"Breast cancer is a largely PREVENTABLE disease, and we reach that good news because of our finding that a large share of recent and current breast cancer in the United States is CERTAINLY due to past medical irradiation of the breasts with x-rays - at all ages, including infancy and childhood. Much of today's radiation dosage is preventable, without any interference with necessary diagnostic radiology, and hence many future breast cancers need not occur." [10]

Epstein concurs with the risks mammograms and x-rays in general pose for the unknowing patient:

"X-rays are carcinogenic. The more X-rays you submit to and the greater the dose, the greater is your risk of cancer... Whatever you may be told, refuse routine mammograms to detect early breast

---

[7] Live on the Laurie Lee Radio Show, 1994

[8] *The Ecologist,* Vol 28, No. 2, March/April 1998, p. 120

[9] Mathe, Prof. George "Scientific Medicine Stymied", *Medicines Nouvelles* (Paris) 1989

[10] Gofman, John W, *Preventing Breast Cancer*, http://www.ratical.com/radiation/ CNR/PBC/indexT.html

cancer, especially if you are pre-menopausal. The X-rays may actually increase your chances of getting cancer.... Very few circumstances, if any, should persuade you to have X-rays taken if you are pregnant. The future risks of leukaemia to your unborn child, not to mention birth defects, are just not worth it." [11]

Breast cancer patients are certainly at risk of developing lung cancer after radiation. In one study of 31 patients who had received radiotherapy for breast cancer, 19 went on to develop a lung cancer, on average, seventeen years later, mostly in the lung located on the same side as the breast that had been irradiated.[12] Some oncologists believe that the lung is especially sensitive to radiation damage, either scar tissue or inflammation – which would tend to argue against high-dose radiotherapy for lung cancer.[13] For Hodgkin's Disease, radiotherapy also poses a risk of breast cancer years later.[14] In rectal cancer, animal studies have demonstrated the descending colon may be especially susceptible to cancer caused by radiation, particularly after surgery, where blood vessels are joined up.[15] The current trend for health departments to promote routine and regular mammograms for early detection of breast cancers is also dangerous nonsense, given the evidence.[16]

The patent failure of modern medicine to halt cancer is now becoming obvious, as the strategies Big Cancer uses to cover up a disaster of its own making are unmasked and exposed for the sham they have become. For instance, in August 1998, the huge MD Anderson Comprehensive Cancer Center in Houston was sued for making the unsubstantiated claim that it cures "well over 50% of people with cancer." Leaflets were deposited in mailboxes throughout the Houston area by MD Anderson in an effort to solicit funds to continue their 'war against cancer.' Misrepresentations and conflicts of interests abound within the cancer industry. For example, the wretched performance of the world's largest 'non-

---

[11] Epstein, Samuel S, *The Politics...*, p.304

[12] *Med. Onc.* 1994; 11:121-5

[13] *Strahl und Onk*, 1995; 171:490-8

[14] *1 Gyne, Ob. et Biol. Repro.* 1995; 24:9-12

[15] *Dis. Colon & Rec.* 1995; 38:152-8

[16] Epstein, Samuel S, *The Politics....* pp. 290, 304, 313, 348-351, 353, etc.

profit' institution, the American Cancer Society (ACS), is examined in the appendix section entitled Conflicts of Interest.

Environmental causations are repeatedly downplayed by Big Cancer, which invariably follows a 'blame the patient' course in explaining the rising causes of cancer. It also partially explains the rise in cancer incidence by alleging that earlier and more accurate detection has inflated the numbers of cancer incidence that were in fact already existing. Another strategy is to state that more people are contracting cancer because they are living longer and therefore stand a statistically higher risk of contracting the disease. Both these allegations are completely false. If age were a factor in cancer, then certainly the Hunzas and other long-lived cultures would be riddled with the disease. Clearly they are not. These strategies serve only to highlight clearly Cancer Inc's extreme reluctance to finger its cousins, Big Industry and Big Food, as the leading cancer felons worldwide today.

Cancer Inc. spares no effort in vilifying and pillorying alternative and non-toxic treatments which have shown a clinical track record of efficacy. Proponents of these treatments have been consistently harassed and defamed, and in certain cases jailed for the stand they have taken on this issue. The unpatentable treatment for cancer we will examine in a moment is not popular with an establishment that has shown itself eminently determined to keep its drug gravy train firmly on the rails.

CANCER - THE NEW APPROACH

In spite of the medical establishment's dictatorial attitude towards protecting their cancer income, huge inroads into conquering cancer were made at the turn of the 1900s by Professor John Beard of Edinburgh University. Beard was no exception in that he received harassment for what he subsequently found. But like many pioneers, he soldiered on nonetheless. John Beard can justifiably be praised for being the individual who broke the back of cancer's mystery and brought its demise forward by many decades.

Beard was an embryologist who was one of the first doctors to study embryonic stem cells, these enigmatic pre-embryonic cells that reside within our body. Beard had noticed that these cells had the ability to develop into the cell structure of any body part, and even into a new embryo, if given the right morphogenetic, hormonal stimulus.

He discovered that in pregnancy, the body uses the hormone estrogen to stimulate these stem cells into rapidly multiplying into a cell mass Beard called 'trophoblast', releasing quantities of human chorionic gonadotrophin (hCG), the hormone later to be detected with a pregnancy test. Beard's thesis stated that these trophoblastic cells have a job to do in pregnancy, namely to etch away part of the uterus wall so that the embryo can attach itself and start to develop.[17] Once this has been achieved, the trophoblastic cells are destroyed around the 56th day of pregnancy when the baby's pancreas comes online and emits its enzymes, which deconstruct the outer coating of the trophoblast, allowing the immune system to clear away the remainder of these cells. Beard had discovered that in the event that the baby's pancreas fails, both the mother and the child die of cancer. In fact, what they die from is an uncontrolled and unregulated proliferation of these trophoblast cells, which now have no pancreatic enzyme 'termination' agents to curtail them.

CANCER AS A ROGUE HEALING PROCESS
Beard found that these stem cells also exist in our body for healing. When we hurt ourselves, our bodies initiate an automatic healing process (survival response) – we know this, and have seen it happen a thousand times. But intriguingly, the healing process commences the same way as with pregnancy trophoblast, namely, the hormone estrogen stimulates our stem cells into producing a trophoblastic 'carpet' of cells which seals off the damaged area and repairs it with cells formed into the cell structure of the bodypart that is being fixed. This healing process is then terminated by pancreatic enzymes upon completion of the task.[18] In the event that we have low levels of these vital pancreatic enzymes, there is no termination agent for the trophoblast in our body and the trophoblast therefore continues to multiply and proliferate

---

[17] The abortion chemical RU486 is designed to prevent this from occurring, thus causing the body to reject the embryo.
[18] Vialls, Joe *Laetrile: Another Suppression Story*, www.livelinks.com/sumeria; *Cancer Control Journal,* Vol. 6. No.1-6

unopposed. The result is an ever expanding mass of trophoblastic cells in our body at the site specific to the original area of damage. Today we call this cell mass a tumour.

Beard discovered that our bodies become depleted of these vital pancreatic enzymes when we eat a diet rich in animal proteins. Without this protection, we become prone to developing cancer if the healing processes that initiate in our bodies are not terminated upon completion of their task. Beard began treating cancer patients to great effect using pancreatic enzymes trypsin and chymotrypsin, as well as other vital nutrients, up until his death around the beginning of World War 1. His theory, as expounded in his papers, was that, by introducing pancreatic enzymes into a cancer patient's body, the enzymes would continue with their job of digesting the outer protein coating of the trophoblast cells, allowing the body to clear away any dangerous trophoblastic proliferation.

We must remember that after Beard's career, medicine began treating cancer patients with Marie Curie's radium and other desperate remedies, causing further trauma, and no doubt generating more trophoblast as a survival response to counter the hurt being done to the body.[19] Beard's work was largely ignored until Ernst T Krebs Jr, a biochemist from Nevada, came across Beard's thesis during his work with enzymes and nutrition.

Krebs was studying those cultures on Earth who did not suffer from cancer. He was aware that men like Albert Schweitzer and explorer Roald Amundsen were coming back from remote areas of the globe reporting that cancer just didn't exist among the populations they had encountered. To the Labrador Eskimos, the Thlinglets, the tribes of Gabon, the Vilcabambans of Ecuador, the Georgian tribes of southern Russia, the Karakorum and Hunzas of eastern Pakistan and the Hopi Indians of Arizona, cancer was unknown – and Krebs was keen to find out why.

He discovered that these peoples differed from westernised populations because they were doing one or all of the following

---

[19] Marie Curie herself was to die from the contamination effects of her own medicine in the 1930s

which Krebs believed resulted in their pronounced and healthy longevity:

- They lived in environments devoid of man-made toxins.
- They ate diets rich in minerals and raw whole foods.
- They ate the dietary compound hydrocyanic acid, a staple of the nitriloside food group, which had been largely eliminated from the diets of Western populations.

Krebs' work on hydrocyanic acid was especially controversial, even as it still is today. The biochemist found that this compound was contained within the apricot seeds of the Hunzas – indeed within all the seeds of the common fruits, excluding citrus, as well as other foods that had largely been cut out of Western diets. The Hunzas were cracking open their apricot pits and consuming the soft seed within along with the pulp of the fruit. In addition, their womenfolk pressed the oil out of the kernels they collected and used it for cooking and cosmetics.

Krebs analysed hydrocyanic acid to discover its life-preserving qualities and reported that when this compound came into contact with trophoblast cells, it selectively killed them by manufacturing two poisons in minute quantities - hydrogen cyanide and benzaldehyde. Krebs also discovered that this reaction did not occur with healthy cells, thus preserving and even nourishing healthy tissue. Research demonstrated that the hydrocyanic acid compound could only be 'unlocked' by beta-glucosidase, a cellular enzyme which, although present throughout the body in minute quantities, was located in huge amounts at the site of trophoblast tumours. The beta-glucosidase contained in the trophoblast cells appeared to 'unlock' the hydrocyanic acid contained in the food to produce hydrogen cyanide and benzaldehyde at the cancer site. The two poisons combined synergistically to produce a super-poison many times more deadly than either substance in isolation. Thus the cancer cell met its chemical death at the hands of this unique compound's selective toxicity.

Krebs ran toxicity studies to determine whether hydrocyanic acid, or Laetrile/amygdalin/Vitamin B17, as the active principal would later become known, was dangerous to the organism if ingested in abnormal quantities. He reported that Vitamin B17 was harmless

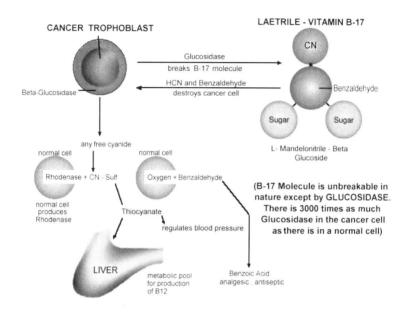

CANCER TROPHOBLAST

LAETRILE - VITAMIN B-17

CN

Glucosidase
breaks B-17 molecule

HCN and Benzaldehyde
destroys cancer cell

Beta-Glucosidase

Benzaldehyde

Sugar   Sugar

L- Mandelonitrile - Beta
Glucoside

any free cyanide

normal cell   normal cell

Rhodenase + CN - Sulf   Oxygen + Benzaldehyde

normal cell
produces
Rhodenase

Thiocyanate

regulates blood pressure

LIVER

metabolic pool
for production
of B12

Benzoic Acid
analgesic ; antiseptic

(B-17 Molecule is unbreakable in
nature except by GLUCOSIDASE.
There is 3000 times as much
Glucosidase in the cancer cell
as there is in a normal cell)

and chemically inert until stimulated by the beta-glucosidase available within cancer cells.

Later other researchers would replicate Krebs' work to confirm these findings. Sheep fed the equivalent of 8-10mg of HCN (hydrogen cyanide) per kilogram per day as linseed meal showed no toxic effects whatsoever. [20] Sheep weighing 66kg were intravenously administered a three-hour dose of 2.7 gms of B17 yielding 300mg of HCN. New Zealand researchers Coop and Blakely reported that *"...at no time during the experiment were even the slightest symptoms observed."* A total of 568mg of HCN was given to a 76kg sheep in the course of an hour. The only symptom the animal showed was *"a general sleepiness for an*

---

[20] Franklin & Reid *Australian Veterinary Journal,* 100:92, 1944

hour". [21] Van der Walt failed to produce chronic poisoning in sheep even after administering 3.2mg HCN/kg daily *for two years.* [22] Worden showed that repeated dosing in rabbits does not produce a cumulative effect and the animal was capable of eliminating excess B17 within two and a half hours.

Other researchers, such as Dr Harold Manner, head of biology at Loyola University, Chicago, ever mindful of the extreme flak Krebs began receiving following the publication of his findings, put further pieces of the cancer puzzle together. Manner began combining Beard's pancreatic enzymes, trypsin and chymotrypsin, with Vitamin A emulsion and B17-Laetrile, and used this protocol with a radical change of diet supplemented with minerals and antioxidants such as Vitamin C and selenium to supercharge the cancer patient to halt the progression of rogue trophoblast and even eliminate it altogether. This procedure was later to form the basis of the nutritional Metabolic Therapy we see practised in the most successful cancer clinics today.

The public and press began showing a marked interest in this controversial research, especially in view of the fact that this new approach to cancer treatment did not involve the use of toxic or radical treatments that were now increasingly becoming viewed as largely useless and 'ethically questionable':

"When President Richard Nixon was deluged with tens of thousands of petitions from ordinary citizens everywhere demanding clinical trials for Laetrile, these demands were forwarded to his cancer advisor, Benno Schmidt... When Schmidt consulted all of his medical colleagues about Laetrile, he found them vehemently opposed to it. But, interestingly enough, as he told reporters later: "I couldn't get anybody to show me scientific proof that the stuff didn't work."" [23]

---

[21] Coop & Blakely *New Zealand Journal of Science & technology*, 28th February 1949, page 277; ibid, 31:(3)1; ibid, February 1950, page 45)
[22] Van der Walt *Veterinary Records*, 52:857, 1940
[23] Heinerman, Dr John *An Encyclopedia of Nature's Vitamins and Minerals*, Prentice Hall, 1998 ISBN 0735200726

In 1973 a three-month trial at the Southern Research Institute in Birmingham, Alabama, intensively researched the therapeutic properties of Laetrile. The institute finally released its findings to the National Cancer Institute which proceeded to announce to the public that once again studies proved that B17-Laetrile had no effect whatsoever in the treatment of cancer. However not all was as it appeared. When the data and protocols from these experiments were subsequently studied in more detail by Dr Dean Burk, one of the National Cancer Institute's founders and head of its Department of Cytochemistry, inconsistencies in the trial protocols began to appear. [24] Researcher G Edward Griffin, whose controversial book *World Without Cancer* broke the Laetrile story to the public in the 1970s, explains:

"Every [Laetrile] *study had been tarnished with the same kind of scientific ineptitude, bias, and outright deception as found in the 1953 MacDonald/Garland California report. Some of these studies openly admitted evidence of anti-cancer effect but hastened to attribute this effect to other causes. Some were toxicity studies only, which means that they weren't trying to see if Laetrile was effective, but merely to determine how much of it was required to kill the patient."* [25]

Despite announcing to the world that Laetrile was useless, the National Cancer Institute, the American Medical Association and the drug cartels looked on with anger as a national grass-roots movement sprang up across America as a result of the many cancer recoveries being reported and attributed to Laetrile and supporting nutrition. It was the '70s and people were distrustful of their government as a result of Watergate and Vietnam. The Committee for Freedom-of-Choice in Cancer Therapy was formed, founding several hundred chapters across America which in turn held public

---

[24] Dean Burk, Ph.D, one of the National Cancer Institute's co-founders, endorsed B17's status as a true vitamin and offered this statement regarding Edward Griffin's *World Without Cancer: "A clear and revolutionary insight into both the science and politics of cancer therapy."* Dr Linus Pauling, the 'father' of Vitamin C and two-time Nobel Laureate, also supported the use of Laetrile (*The New England Journal of Medicine*, 8th July 1982)

[25] Griffin, G Edward *World Without Cancer*, ibid.

meetings, press conferences and pressured state legislative committees into calling for the 'legalisation' of Vitamin B17.

The federal government eventually persuaded the cancer industry to test Laetrile, which they did – without the pancreatic enzymes and other supporting co-factors required to break down the cancer cell. Of course the trials failed and the results – or lack of them – were subsequently reported, the summary declaring that Laetrile has no anti-cancer benefit whatsoever. Meanwhile, other cancer industry-appointed scientists, such as Dr Kanematsu Sugiura, Dr Elizabeth Stockert and Dr Lloyd Schoen, were using the correct protocols at Memorial Sloan-Kettering and achieving startling results, as others would around the world in the years to come.

But even these results were mis-reported, and once again B17 was 'tossed under the bus' with Memorial Sloan-Kettering's incredible conclusion: *"These results allow no definite conclusion supporting the anti-cancer activity of Laetrile."*[26]

This did not stop many physicians across America and later the world from implementing this therapy into their treatments of cancer patients. Many of these professionals received constant harassment at the hand of the medical authorities, who accused them of practising quackery and treating their patients with an 'unappoved drug' which contained the dangerous 'cyanide'. Gradually, through persistent and at times downright paranoid propaganda, the little yellow apricot became a natural-born killer in the eyes of many. Interestingly, the establishment proved dismal in the consistency of its opposition, focusing on "cyanide – what are you crazy?!" but failing to pillory Vitamin B12 as a 'deadly agent', containing as it does the cyanide radical also (Vitamin B12 is known as cyanocobalamin).

Philip Binzel MD, a doctor who retrained to treat his cancer patients with this nutritional therapy, foregoing the dangers of toxic chemotherapy and radiation treatments, highlights in his book *Alive and Well* the problem many doctors were having with an inherent lack of knowledge on nutrition:

---

[26] Griffin, G Edward, ibid.

"Most of my first patients were those who had all of the surgery, radiation and chemotherapy they could tolerate and their tumors were still growing. I did for these patients the best I knew to do.

My biggest problem at the time was understanding nutrition. <u>In four years of medical school, one year of Family Practice residency, I had not had even one lecture on nutrition.</u>" [emphasis mine] [27]

Binzel's book catalogues the repeated harassment he received at the hands of the Ohio State Medical Board and the Food & Drug Administration over his use of Laetrile and nutritional co-factors for his cancer patients. Binzel's incredible story of amazing tumour regressions and eliminations amid the backdrop of draconian treatment at the hands of his peers is typical of the rollercoaster ride many courageous doctors underwent in order to bring the truth of wellness to their suffering patients.

Even the Food & Drug Administration had its defectors. June de Spain, one of its pharmacologists and toxicologists, wrote *The Little Cyanide Cookbook*, in which she dispels the 'deadly-cyanide-in-its-natural-form' myth and lays out hundreds of diets containing the essential nitriloside factor. De Spain sums up her own findings on the back cover of her book:

"Because of its unique molecular structure, this compound releases cyanide only at the cancer site, thus destroying cancer cells while nourishing non-cancer tissue. Those populations in the world which eat these vitamin-rich foods simply do not get cancer – and they live to be much older than those who subsist on the typical modern diet.

Cyanide in minute quantities and in the proper food forms, instead of being poisonous, actually is an essential component of

---

[27] Binzel, P E *Alive & Well,* American Media, 2000 (available through Credence at www.credence.org)

normal body chemistry. Vitamin B12, for instance, contains cyanide in the form of cyanocobalamin." [28]

Other doctors around the world were doing their own research, such as Dr Hans Nieper, former Director of the Department of Medicine at Silbersee Hospital in Hanover, Germany: During a visit to the United States in 1972, Dr Nieper told reporters: *"After more than twenty years of such specialised work, I have found non-toxic nitrilosides – that is, Laetrile – far superior to any other known cancer treatment or preventative. In my opinion, it is the only existing possibility for the ultimate control of cancer."*

In Canada, Dr N R Bouziane, former Director of Research Laboratories at St Jeanne D'Arc Hospital in Montreal, published his repeated successes in treating cancers with nutrition, which were written up in the medical literature, including the *Cancer News Journal*, Jan/April 1971, p.20, under the article heading "The Laetrile Story".

In the Philippines, Dr Manuel Navarro, former Professor of Medicine and Surgery at the University of Santo Tomas, Manila, and an internationally recognised cancer researcher with over 100 major scientific papers to his credit, treated terminally ill cancer patients with Laetrile for over 25 years. He stated in the *Cancer News Journal*: *"It is my carefully considered clinical judgement, as a practising oncologist and researcher in this field, that I have obtained most significant and encouraging results with the use of Laetrile-amygdalin in the treatment of terminal cancer patients..."* [29]

In Mexico, Dr Ernesto Contreras, one of the country's leading medical specialists in nutritional treatment for cancer for over 30 years, remarks of B17-Laetrile's action with extreme terminal cancer cases: *"The palliative action* [the ability of a substance to improve the comfort of a patient] *is in about 60% of the cases.*

---

[28] De Spain, June *The Little Cyanide Cookbook*, American Media, 2000. For superb dietary ideas, see also Day, Phillip *Food For Thought*, Credence, 2000 (also available at the Credence web-site at www.credence.org)
[29] *Cancer News Journal,* Jan/April 1971, pp.19-21

Frequently, enough to be significant, I see arrest of the disease or even regression in some 15% of the very advanced cases."[30]

Ernesto's son Francisco Contreras continues the work today after his father's retirement. Francisco is author of *The Hope of Living Cancer Free* in which he lays out the protocols his clinic has used to marvellous success in treating thousands of patients since 1963.[31]

In Italy, Professor Etore Guidetti, of the University of Turin Medical School, announced startling results with Laetrile in successfully combating many types of cancer, including cervix, breast, uterus and rectum. After a speech, an American doctor rose in the audience, challenging the Italian professor that Laetrile had been found to be worthless in the United States. Dr Guidetti was abrupt and dismissive: *"I care not what was determined in the United States. I am merely reporting what I saw in my own clinic."*[32]

This chapter sets the premise for the technical information that follows, as we work through the scientific proof and rationale for metabolic therapy.

---

[30] These are cases receiving a 100% death-rate prognosis, given up as hopeless by orthodox medicine. The fact that any of these survive *at all* is astonishing in itself. Dr Contreras' words were reported in the *Cancer News Journal*, Vol 9, No 3. Source: The Arlin J. Brown Inf. Center, Inc, PO Box 251, Fort Belvoir, VA 22060. 703 451 8638. Tel: 540 752 9511. E mail: cancerinfo@webtv.net

[31] Contreras, Francisco *The Hope of Living Cancer Free*, Siloam Press, 1999. A detailed overview of the nutritional therapy practised in many cancer clinics today. Contreras also examines the psychological and spiritual factors so important in assisting a patient in overcoming their illness and helping them through the healing process.

[32] *Cancer News Journal*, ibid.

ERNST KREBS SPEAKS

Taken from a 1974 speech presented before the Second Annual Cancer Convention at the Ambassador Hotel in Los Angeles, California.

"It is certainly a pleasure to be here at the Second Annual Convention of the Cancer Control Society - an outgrowth, as you know, of the International Association of Cancer Victims and Friends.

As I look back through the years marking the emergence of these two fine societies, I can recall the number of miraculous victories we have had in those intervening years; that it is as true today as it was eleven years ago that Laetrile, Vitamin B17, is the first and last final hope in the prophylacsis in therapy of cancer in man and animals. The reason for this is that Laetrile is a vitamin. It is the 17th of the B vitamins.

We hear a great deal about its use in terminal cancer, but the time to start with Vitamin B17 is now before the disease becomes clinical. The time to start is the same with any matter of adequate nutrition and that is right now. You may start now by commencing to eat the seeds of all common fruits that you eat. Apricot and peach seeds contain almost 2 percent of Vitamin B17 by weight. The apple seed, although very small, is equally rich in Vitamin B17 - so are the seeds of prunes, plums, cherries, and nectarines. The only common fruits on the hemisphere that lack nitrilosidic seeds are the citrus fruits. This lack has come about by artificial cultivation, by breeding and hybridization, since the seeds of citrus fruits on the African continent still contain Vitamin B17.

Two more rich sources of Vitamin B17 are the simple cereal millet and buckwheat. Macadamia nuts, although expensive and exotic, are very rich in Vitamin B17 and so are bamboo shoots, mung beans, lima beans, butter beans and certain strains of garden peas. But for convenience, the simple source for your Vitamin B17 are the seeds of the common fruit.

We know something about the prophylactic dose of Vitamin B17. For example, we know the Hunzas represent a population that has been cancer-free for over 900 years of its existence. This population has a natural diet which supplies on the average between 50 to 75 milligrams of Vitamin B17 a day.

Hunzaland is a land that has sometimes been described as the 'place where the apricot is king.' The Hunzakuts eat fresh apricots for the three months they are in season and for the remainder of the year they eat dried apricots. They never eat a dried apricot without enclosing the seed. This supplies them with better than the average of 50 to 75 milligrams of Vitamin B17 a day.

There are many of us in the western world who don't ingest this amount of Vitamin B17 in the course of an entire year. As a result we're in the midst of a fulminating deficiency of Vitamin B17 or nitriloside, the anti-neoplastic vitamin. Its absence from our diets accounts for the fact that cancer within our population has reached such a pandemisity as to account for its occurrence in one in every three American families. The occurrence is probably much greater than that because it is very late in its development when the cancer is detected. Many who develop cancer are killed by accident or intercurrent diseases before the malignant process has become sufficiently advanced to cause them to have it diagnosed.

Cancer is a chronic, metabolic disease - that is obvious. It isn't an infectious disease, which is caused by bacteria or viruses. It is a disease that is metabolic in origin. A metabolic disease is a disease that is wedded to our utilization of food. Most metabolic diseases have as their basis the deficiency of specific vitamins and minerals.

Let me give you a categorical or axiomatic truth to take with you - one that is totally uncontradictable, scientifically, historically and in every other way. This is, that no chronic or metabolic disease in the history of medicines has ever been prevented or cured except by factors normal to the diet or normal to the animal economy. There have been many erstwhile fatal and devastating diseases that now have become virtually unknown. They have been prevented and cured by ingesting the dietary factors and thereby preventing the deficiencies which accounted for these diseases.

The one with which you are probably most familiar is scurvy - a fatal disease that killed mankind by the thousands; a disease that would sometimes wipe out an entire polar expedition. Scurvy accounted for about 50 percent mortality among the Crusaders. It is a disease that can be totally prevented and cured with Vitamin C or ascorbic acid - a factor normal to an adequate diet. As you know so well from your school days, Great Britain acquired the dominion of the seas by discovering that through adding lime or other citrus juices to the provisions of the British mariners, the curse of scurvy from the British sea power was removed. Therefore Britain competitively gained the ascendancy on the seas. Prior to the incorporation of Vitamin C into their diets, it wasn't uncommon for three-fourths of the crew to become seriously ill by the end of a voyage and then those who didn't die would mysteriously recover after hitting shore because they would have access to fresh fruits and vegetables rich in Vitamin C.

Then we have pernicious anemia, which had a mortality rate of 98 or 99 percent and no medical modality under the sun could touch it. Arsenic and its salts, strychnine, iron and hundreds of other remedies were tried but to no avail until the researchers Drs. Murphy, Shipple and Minot commenced their classical studies on the relationship of pernicious anemia to dietary deficiency.

While working at the University of California they discovered a very simple remedy for preventing and curing this disease. They simply said to their patients, "Go down to your butcher shop and get a quarter pound of fresh liver. Grind it up and take a tablespoon everyday and take the quarter pound and cook it very lightly and just singe the surface and use this as a ration for three days." And when the patients followed this advice without exception, those with pernicious anemia made complete recoveries. Despite this, these men were censored by the Medical Establishment at the time and were criticized for engaging in what was alleged to be medical quackery.

The argument was, how could respectable doctors advise people with a disease that has a 99 percent mortality rate to ignore all of the established drugs of medical science and go down to the butcher shop and buy some raw liver and take this and expect this to cure a disease that nothing else had cured. Well, raw liver did cure the disease and raw liver prevented it. As the chemistry of raw liver was studied it was discovered that the factors responsible were Vitamin B12[33] and Folic Acid. So Vitamin B12 and Folic Acid are now a part of our normal dietary experience.

And so in 1974, the uninformed, the unimaginative and some of the illiterate are concerned with what to them is a preposterous idea that by eating the seeds of fruit you can prevent a disease that carries a mortality rate almost as high as that once carried by pernicious anemia. But scientific truth isn't dependent upon credibility or lack of it. The scientific reality either is or it isn't. And this is the scientific reality - that the seeds of all common fruits (except citrus) contain Vitamin B17, an anti-cancer vitamin. If we ingest proper quantities of this vitamin either in the pure form or through ingesting the nitrilosidic foods, we will be able to prevent this disease just as surely as we are able to prevent scurvy by the use of Vitamin C or pernicious anemia by the use of Vitamin B12.

There was another disease that had a metabolic or chronic nature and this was pellagra. At one time it was so endemic in certain parts of the world, particularly the American South-East, that there were entire hospitals given to the treatment of pellagrins.

The great Sir William Osler, in his *Principles and Practices of Medicine*, written at the turn of this century, said of pellagra, *"I was at Lenoir, North Carolina during one winter and I visited the Lenoir home for the colored insane and there 75 percent of the inmates died from the disease. It ran rampant through this institution and convinced me beyond any doubt that pellagra is a virus that is infectious."*

And then came the fine works of the United States Public Health Service surgeon, Dr Goldberger, who showed conclusively that the occurrence of pellagra was related to a deficiency of fresh green material in the diet. So Dr Goldberger approached this problem

---

[33] Like B17, Vitamin B12 also contains the cyanide radical, hence its name, cyanocobalamin

first by the use of brewer's yeast, which would completely prevent and cure pellagra. Further studies then showed that the factor in brewer's yeast that was most determinate of this effect was niacin, Vitamin B3.

So another fatal chronic metabolic disease found total resolution and cure through factors normal to the regular diet of the animal economy. We know that cancer is no exception to this great generalization which to date has known no exception. That is, that every chronic or metabolic disease that will ever be controlled by man must be controlled by means that are a part of the biological experience of the organism. Chronic and metabolic diseases can never be controlled, prevented or cured by factors [drugs] foreign to the biological experience of the organism.

Dr Thomas of the Sloan-Kettering Institute in a recent article in *Science* said, *"I'm thankful that my liver works without my knowledge. I do not have the brains to commence to do one millionth of what my liver does. These things are automatic. So I swallow the food and this infinitely complex machinery takes care of itself."*

We could spend years telling you about this magnificent machinery and we still wouldn't touch the surface of this infinite ocean. We do know that there is nothing that we can do to improve upon it. We do know that in the history of medicine there never has been found anything foreign to the indwelling requirements of this machinery that will do the living organism any good. And we can go further to say there has never in the history of medicine been found anything foreign to the indwelling machinery of this infinitely complex system that will not harm the organism. There isn't such a thing as a factor foreign to the biological experience that is not harmful to the organism.

There is nothing we can add to our air, water and food to improve it. The most we can do is to look at some of our devitalized food and hopefully attempt to replace that which was capriciously removed from it in the process of food refining, manipulation or cooking. There is absolutely nothing that we can add to that food to improve it. These things are basic.

There isn't any chemical or drug that medical science could suggest that would make us healthier or better adjusted or wiser or give us hope for a longer life. There isn't a single drug or molecule in nature that can accomplish this unless that molecule exists in normal food. And this probably explains one of the reasons why there is so much resistance to Laetrile, B17.

The application of this science brings us face to face with a lot of things we do not like to face. We have become over-civilized. We are inclined in our delusory thinking to feel that there must be a magic 'out', that there must be a simple way, a short cut, that somehow or other medical science or some other man-made force beyond our comprehension will do for us those things we must do for ourselves. And it is slowly dawning on us, perhaps too slowly, that this thinking is fraudulent, that it is unsound.

It isn't in the field of cancer alone where we see this form of charlatanism or quackery. We see it in the area of the human mind - the futile attempts to spare man from the realities that surround him. Above all to spare him from the fact that he is accountable to himself and to his God and that there is no short cut in this accountability.

It's real at the physical level. And when we are eating less than adequate food, we know better. And when we continue we are engaged in sin, this is the basis for practically all of our physical and mental and spiritual difficulties. We had better be realistic about it. We have these difficulties because we don't do the right things. And when we fail in view of our knowledge now to take Vitamin B17, this is a sin against our physical nature. And when we develop cancer we will receive the results of this transgression in the old fashion Biblical sense that the "wages of sin are death."

If you are not getting Vitamin B17 in your food, the best way to get it is in the pure form. If you have cancer, the most important single consideration is to get the maximum amount of Vitamin B17 into your body in the shortest period of time. This is secondary to the medical skill involved in administering it, which is relatively minimal. Then very often there are many supportive measures that are taken in the management of the cancer patient such as the use of materials to build up the blood and immune system, to raise or lower the blood pressure or to relieve the pain.

Pancreatic enzymes and vegetable enzymes are part of the supportive theory. You have the papaya melons as the source of the enzyme papain and pineapple as a source of the enzyme bromelain. The demasking effect of these enzymes against the pericellular layer of the malignant cell is something very concrete in the immunology of cancer. Now I prefer, rather than advising the use of bromelain or papaya tablets, that the individual seeking these enzymes get them directly from the fresh ripe pineapple and papaya fruit. As much as half a pineapple a day should be ingested.

This is the way to go. You have nothing to lose by eating fresh pineapple and papaya melons. Nothing to lose by eating millet, the seeds of all the common fruits and whole fresh foods.

Dietary deficiencies arrive primarily from eating less than whole food. This is why the American federal and state governments have made mandatory the artificial enrichment of white flour. Look at any loaf of white bread or white flour that has been enriched by the addition of crystalline Vitamin B1, Vitamin B2, niacin, iron and all the rest. What a commentary on the stupidity of our civilization that we put good food through a process that deprives it of its essential nutrients and then we are compelled by government mandate to restore to this food some of the things that have been processed out. One of the most critical factors is removed and that is wheat germ, which contains Vitamin E and the polyunsaturated fatty acids. It would not be necessary to take it in supplementation if our foods were not manipulated in a way which removes these factors.

Now something about supplementation in addition to the Vitamin B17. We can't think in terms of just one vitamin. We get an adequate diet by eating as wide a variety of whole natural foods as possible and as close to their growing period as we can possibly obtain them.

38

There are Laetrile therapists who recommend two or three grams of ascorbic acid or Vitamin C in conjunction with the Laetrile program. This is a very moderate recommendation and we can all take up to seven or eight grams of Vitamin C without any problems. This is about the same amount as animals such as the gorilla, on a pound-to-pound basis, ingest - between five to six grams of Vitamin C a day in their normal habitat. Incidentally, the gorilla in its natural habitat eats about 100 to 125 milligrams of Vitamin B17 every day too. Like the population of Hunzaland, these gorillas are free of cancer.

Bears are also free of cancer in their normal habitat. In the wild, bears don't develop cancer. In the San Diego Zoo, there was a cage of about ten bears and out of the ten, seven of them developed cancer. To some this was a sign that some mysterious bear cancer virus was on the loose, but it wasn't that at all. In the wild state, bears are omnivores and they eat a lot of wild nitrilosidic berries. Almost all wild fruits are nitrilosidic.

Keep in mind how far we have drifted from the dietary requirements of the machinery we possess. The fruit we eat today is the product of years of manipulation and cultivation for lushness and abundance and so forth, so the meat to that fruit is free of Vitamin B17. To meet our indwelling needs of Vitamin B17 we must either eat the fruit seed in reasonable quantities or begin supplementing our diet with Vitamin B17 tablets. We can't of course do that at present [due to legislation], but we hope to see before very long Vitamin B17 available so that we can prevent cancer in the same way we prevent scurvy.

Several new books are coming out on Laetrile. Both are written by non-medical men: *World Without Cancer* by Edward Griffin and *Vitamin B17: Forbidden Weapon Against Cancer* by Mike Culbert. We are all laymen in the field of cancer. There are laymen in the Laetrile movement who know more about cancer than some of our most prestigious experts in our most prestigious institutions. These laymen know enough about it to keep alive and not die from it. So you're a pretty rotten expert if you know so little about it as to succumb from it or have your family succumb from it.

We have many case histories of people who have been helped by Laetrile. Both Alicia Buttons and Mary Henderson were terminal with oral pharyngeal cancer that has a mortality rate of 98-99 percent even in early diagnosis. Both made remarkable recoveries with Laetrile under the guidance of Dr Hans Nieper in Germany.

You know we have been meeting for ten or eleven years and you've been hearing this story. Each time after the meeting you had 360 days to go home and read newspapers, American Cancer Society technical journals, Boiler Plate and so forth. In those ten years they haven't told you anything against Laetrile that makes any sense. You can be pretty sure they don't have anything against Laetrile because these people are very uninhibited and the area in which they are most uninhibited is the area of simple lying.

If you have any questions about Laetrile, the more critical the better because we are dealing with solid science. We are dealing with a science that admits that there is no rational alternative in the ten years that have passed since these meetings began. Nothing has come about which does anything except make more obvious the fact that Laetrile, Vitamin B17, is the answer to cancer."

ABOUT THIS AUTHOR

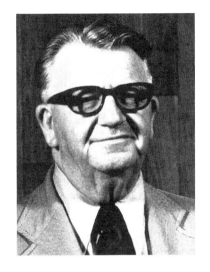

Ernst Theodor Krebs Jr. was born in Carson City, Nevada. He attended medical college in Philadelphia from 1938-41 and received his AB degree from the University of Illinois in 1942. He was a graduate student at the University of California Berkeley (UCB) from 1943-45 and researched in pharmacy from 1942-45. Krebs and his father, Ernst Krebs Sr. MD, are also credited with pioneering the medical applications for Vitamin B15 or pangamic acid, a nutrient largely embargoed by the medical establishment. During the pre-war years, Krebs concentrated his studies on the knowledge and use of enzymes, including bromelain, chymotrypsin, trypsin and papain, in the treatment of cancer. Both Krebs and his father are widely recognised today as the pioneers of Vitamin B17, otherwise known as amygdalin or Laetrile, in its role in the treatment of cancer, although the substance was in use as a medicinal aid much earlier.

THE HUNZAS
by Phillip Day
Credence Research

Upon embarking on a study of longevity, you don't get very far into the project before you come into contact with the Hunzas. This isolated people of Northeastern Pakistan, located in the Himalayan foothill valleys, were not discovered until the 1920s, when the British Army traversed the mountain passes and came into contact with one of humankind's longevity miracles for the very first time. One practitioner who went with them was Dr Robert McCarrison (later Sir Robert McCarrison), who was able to document in some detail the astonishing culture he discovered.

The society the army engineers found was open, warm, friendly and religious and had a tremendous sense of community. One of the things McCarrison noticed immediately was the astonishing lack of diseases and the fine condition of the people. In their indigenous, isolated environment, the Hunzas exhibited near perfect physical and mental health. There was no sign of cancer, heart disease, diabetes, ulcers, colitis, diverticulosis, high blood pressure or childhood ailments. Neither was there any juvenile delinquency or crime. Respect for elders and age was ubiquitous and the tribe's sense of community made it clear to all members that if one was to succeed, all had to succeed. The teamwork with which the Hunzas executed their daily chores was very evident in their happiness, peace of mind and conspicuous lack of strife. The Hunzas had no police, no jails, no judges and no doctors or hospitals.

Their teeth were in the finest condition - perfect dental arches full of even, white teeth with no disfiguration, dental caries or other tarnishments common to the industrialised societies. Many of their population were later estimated to be older than 100, fathering children at 100-plus, with some of the most vital apparently surviving to 150 and beyond. Hunza womenfolk too were of the finest condition. No birth problems were observed and those ladies of 80 looked the equivalent of 40, with fresh and remarkably unblemished complexions.

McCarrison, later to become Director of Research on Nutrition in India and Chairman of the Post-Graduate Medical Education Committee at Oxford University, was so taken by these people that he spent years of his life uncovering the Hunzas' health secrets. He later wrote: *"These people are unsurpassed by any other race in perfection of physique. They are long-lived, vigorous in youth and age, capable of great endurance and enjoy remarkable freedom from disease in general."* [34]

Renee Taylor too studied the Hunzas and was told by their King, the Mir: *"The idleness of retirement is a much greater enemy in life than work. One must never retire from something, one must retire to something."* [35]

The Hunza workload was prodigious. It was common, researcher Roger French reports, for a Hunza to walk the 200km return trip to Gilgit in neighbouring Pakistan, carrying a heavy load over mountain passes and dangerous terrain without any stops for rest other than meal breaks. The men regularly played vigorous games, including volleyball and polo. In a strenuous game of volleyball, the young men, aged 16 to 50, would play against the elders, who were well over 70 and, as observed in one game, included a man thought to be 125 years old. Hunza polo was ferocious and without rules and there were often teeth knocked out. As the Mir remarked: *"The men of 100 felt no more fatigue than the men of 20."* [36]

McCarrison got to the bottom of the Hunzas' success and roundly attributed it to super-nutrition and the absence of a toxic, industrially polluted environment. Hunza water was found to be highly mineralised, with a spectrum of nutrients derived from fresh mountain streams and glaciers. The Hunzas also irrigated with this mineral-rich mixture, greatly benefiting the crops that were subsequently harvested and eaten. McCarrison also noted that the Hunzas ate a high percentage of their foods raw and as close to nature as possible. Biochemist Ernst Krebs, along with other

[34] **French, Roger** *The Man Who Lived in Three Centuries*, Natural Health Society of Australia, 2000, p. 29
[35] **Taylor, Renee** *Hunza Health Secrets*, Keats Publishing, 1964
[36] French, Roger, ibid. p.30

researchers, would also remark that the Hunzas, proud farmers of apricots, always consumed the seeds (kernels) of their fruits along with the pulp. This practice is widely condemned in Western societies today because of a supposed danger of cyanide poisoning (more details in a later chapter).

McCarrison set out to prove how diet was a major contributor to the Hunzas' success by taking rats and feeding them a staple Hunza diet – fresh fruits and vegetables, dried fruits, legumes, whole-grain foods and goat's cheese and butter. Meat was a rarity, and the meat and dairy components of their diet were low, in contrast to Westernised diets today.

McCarrison's Hunza rats were extremely long-lived and almost completely free of disease. Their condition was sleek, their childbirth easy and free of complications and the young ones were gentle, good-natured and healthy.

McCarrison then fed another sample of rats on the diet of the poor of the Bengal/Madras region: lots of rice, old pulses and vegetables, condiments and a little milk, together with city water. As described in his book, *Studies in Deficiency Diseases*, McCarrison's Bengal/Madras rats were not happy rodents. The list of diseases afflicting them included diseases of the ear, nose and throat, lungs and upper respiratory tract, gastrointestinal diseases, skin diseases, reproductive problems, cancer of the blood and lymph, heart disease and edema.

Finally McCarrison fed a third sample of rats the same diet consumed by the working-class Englishman of the day: refined, white bread and sugar, margarine, sweetened tea, boiled vegetables, tinned meats and jams. The same rash of diseases as previously reported with the Bengal/Madras group broke out among the rats, this time with severe additional complications; namely nervous diseases and pronounced delinquency among the rodents, which bit their attendants constantly and finally, by the 16th day of the experiment, began turning upon their own, killing each other and cannibalising the weaker among them. McCarrison's summary was succinct:

"I know of nothing so potent in producing ill-health as improperly constituted food. It may therefore be taken as a law of life, infringement of which shall surely bring its own penalties, that the single greatest factor in the acquisition of health <u>is perfectly constituted food</u>. Given the will, we have the power to build in every nation a people more fit, more vigorous and competent; a people with longer and more productive lives, and with more physical and mental stamina than the world has ever known." [37]
[emphasis mine]

---

[37] **French, Roger** *The Man Who Lived in Three Centuries*, Natural Health Society of Australia, 2000, p. 32

THE NITRILOSIDES IN PLANTS AND ANIMALS
Nutritional and Therapeutic Implications
by Ernst T Krebs Jr.
John Beard Memorial Foundation

Since the principal objective of this presentation is a study of the clinical use of the Laetriles (nitrilosides), because these substances yield nascent HCN [hydrogen cyanide/prussic acid] when they undergo enzymatic hydrolysis *in vivo,* it will be helpful if one begins with a general study of the nitrilosides in plants and animals.

A nitriloside is a naturally occurring or synthetic compound which, upon hydrolysis by a beta-glucosidase, yields a molecule of a non-sugar, or aglycone, a molecule of free hydrogen cyanide, and one or more molecules of a sugar or its acid. There are approximately 14 naturally occurring nitrilosides distributed in over 1200 species of plants. Nitrilosides are found in all plant phyla from *Thallopliyta* to *Sperimatophyta*.

The nitrilosides specifically considered in this paper are 1-mandelonitrile-beta-diglucoside (amygdalin) and its hydrolytic products; l-para-hydroxymandelonitrile-beta-glucoside (dhurrin); methylethyl-ketone-cyanohydrin-beta-glucoside (lotaustralin); and acetone- cyanohydrin-beta-glucoside (linamarin). All of these compounds are hydrolyzed to free HCN, one or more sugars and a non-sugar or aglycone. For the purposes of this study, they may be considered as physiologically and pharmacologically identical and varying essentially only in the percent of free HCN they produce upon hydrolysis by beta-glucosidase.

The concentration of nitrilosides in plants varies widely and ranges from small traces to as much as 30,000 mg/kg in some of the common pasture grasses (in the dry state). There is no evidence that animals synthesize nitrilosides under normal conditions. The metabolism of all the higher animals, and most of the invertebrates as well, involves the hydrolysis of plant-derived nitrilosides ingested in the plant components of the diet. This hydrolysis is produced by beta-glucosidase occurring in the gastro-intestinal tract and produced in various tissues of the animal. The enzyme occurring in the intestinal tract is produced by various bacteria or microflora. When the enzyme so produced or that enzyme existing in the organs acts to hydrolyze the nitrilosides to free HCN, sugar and a non-sugar moiety, the CN ion released is detoxified or converted by an enzyme normally occurring in the organism and known as *rhodanese* or thiosulfate transulfurase. The product of such conversion is thiocyanate, a compound found in the tissues of all vertebrates, many invertebrates and a number of plants.

It is one of the objectives of this report to survey extensively but not intensively the indispensable but long-overlooked role of the nitrilosides in the plant and animal kingdoms. The material utilized for this paper comprises, to a large extent, an abstract of a book now in preparation on the subject. The latter carries a bibliography in excess of 3,000 titles. It is not possible in this report to supply an adequate bibliography. We have therefore limited the references in this paper, as a rule, to isolated or specific experimental observations; and we have omitted the citation of reference sources for data that are commonplace or unquestioned facts in the universe of the relevant expert. For this reason, statements undocumented here may often appear extraordinary to a reader not intimately acquainted with sophisticated data derived from disciplines often distant from his own. For example, even to experts in animal husbandry, agriculture, pharmacology, and toxicology, it may come as an almost unbelievable statement that cattle, in the course of grazing, may daily ingest grasses containing as much as 30,000 mg/kg of nitriloside (carrying over 2.0 grams of derivable HCN) over a period of years without discernible effect. The grasses involved have, however, been repeatedly assayed by reliable and universally accepted techniques and the quantities ingested by sheep and cattle have been repeatedly and carefully measured. The results have been duly published in acceptable journals over the world.

NITRILOSIDES AND NITRILES
IN TERMS OF BIOLOGICAL EXPERIENCE
Nitrilosides are produced by, and HCN enters into the metabolism of, members of the plant kingdom extending from bacteria, moulds and fungi to the common fruits - apricots, peaches, cherries, berries, and the like - comprising the *Rosaceae* and extending

through the *Leguminosae* - lima beans, vetch, pulses, clovers - to the *Graminae* with over eighty grasses of the latter family carrying one or more specific nitrilosides.

No area of the earth that supports vegetation lacks nitriloside-containing plants. Over 30 per cent of *all* tropical plants, edible or inedible by man or animals, contain a nitriloside. From the nitriloside-rich salmon-berry, cloud-berry or buffalo-berry (*Rubus spectabilis*) growing on the Arctic tundra and the arrow-grass growing in arctic marshes and supplying the major fodder for the caribou, to the cassava or manioc - the bread of the tropics - plants extraordinarily rich in nitriloside, and serving as food for man and animals, are found in abundance. All life on earth participates directly or indirectly in the chain of nitriloside metabolism. In terms of living forms, the nitrilosides appear as ubiquitous in time as they do in space. There is some evidence that life on earth commenced in conjunction with hydrogen cyanide.

A glance at the vegetation about us almost anywhere will disclose nitriloside-containing plants. The common weed and fodder, Johnson-grass, often carries 15,000 mg/kg or more of nitriloside. A similar concentration is found in Sudan-grass, Velvet grass, white clover, the Yetches, buckwheat, the millets, alfalfa or lucerne, lima beans, even some strains of green or garden peas, the quinces, all species of the passion-flower. The seeds as well as the leaves and roots of the peaches and various cherries are but a few of the natural sources of this essentially non-toxic water-soluble factor.

METABOLIC ROLE
Though the nitrilosides are plant-produced, we are interested here only in their metabolic role in the animal kingdom. We know that they account largely if not exclusively for all the thiocyanate found in the tissue and body fluids of animals. Thiocyanate is found in the serum, urine, sweat, saliva and tears of man and other mammals. Thiocyanate, as well as its natural precursor, the HCN derived from dietary nitrilosides, supply the cyanide ion for the nitrilization of the precursor of vitamin B12 (hydro[xy]cobalamin) to vitamin B12 (cyanocobalamin).

Upon hydrolysis in the intestinal tract of man or animals, the nitriloside exerts a variable antibiotic effect through the action of the freed hydrogen cyanide and, in the case of some nitrilosides such as amygdalin or dhurrin, through the antiseptic action of benzaldehyde or p-hydroxybenzaldehyde aglycone. The latter from Johnson-grass, before and after oxidation to a benzoic acid, is about 30 times more antiseptic (in terms of the phenol coefficient) than ordinary benzaldehyde or benzoic acid. It is now experimentally established that *only* those nitrile compounds that are hydrolyzed to *free hydrogen cyanide* lend themselves to the formation, through rhodanese in the presence of utilizable sulfur, of thiocyanate.

EXCRETION

After metabolism in the animal body, most of the HCN moiety is eliminated as thiocyanate in the urine with possibly some being eliminated in the feces. In man, a small percentage of the nitriloside-derived HCN may be excreted through the lungs and even in the urine. In rabbits, the administration of one nitriloside (amygdalin) has been reported as resulting in the elimination of traces of the unchanged nitriloside in the urine. Sorghum and other plants involved in cyanogenesis associated with the synthesis of nitriloside are known to emit a small percentage of free HCN.

In the case of nitrilosides with an acetone aglycone or an ethylmethyl-ketone aglycone, the ketone aglycones as well as the sugar moiety are probably fully metabolized to carbon dioxide and water with the HCN residue contributing to the production of thiocyanate, some of which may be eliminated from the body in the urine and feces with the remainder persisting as part of the normal "cyanide metabolic pool".

EVIDENCE FOR BETA-GLUCOSIDASE
IN ANIMAL TISSUES

The enzyme beta-glucosidase is found in especially high concentrations in the liver, spleen, kidney and intestinal mucosa in animals. Since HCN is eliminated as thiocyanate and since only nitriles split to free HCN can experience thiocyanate conversion by rhodanese in the presence of a source of sulfur, the fact that ingested nitrilosides increase the level of thiocyanate in the body fluids proves that they have been hydrolyzed to free HCN. This hydrolysis is enzymatically accomplished only by a beta-glucosidase.

Nitrilosides are also hydrolyzed to free HCN when injected into the peritoneal cavity of the rabbit. The fluid in this area apparently is lacking in rhodanese activity, since free HCN has been observed in the peritoneal fluid of rabbits following injections of large doses of amygdalin. Extensive studies have also been published on the hydrolysis of nitrilosides to free HCN by the rumenal microflora of sheep.

EVIDENCE FOR OCCURRENCE OF
RHODANESE IN VERTEBRATES
The detoxification of HCN as thiocyanate was first observed by S. Lang in 1894, and the enzymic aspects were first studied in 1933 by K. Lang who gave the name *rhodanese* to the enzyme concerned. Since thiocyanate is some hundred times or so less toxic than HCN, the rhodanese reaction is a true detoxification.

It appears that the concentration or activity of rhodanese in the tissues of animals varies directly with the normal nitriloside content of the general diet characterizing each species. The livers of rats, rabbits and cows appear to be more active than those of monkeys, men, dogs, and cats in descending order. Rhodanese activity is as widely distributed in living forms as are the nitrilosides. Both have been found in forms as diverse as fish, squid, insects and plants. The enzyme has been isolated in crystalline form by Sorbo and a substantial literature on it has developed. The action of rhodanese is highly specific. It is limited not merely to nitriles but only to those nitrilosides which surrender free HCN ions upon hydrolysis.

The administration of rhodanese has been found to protect experimental animals from doses of cyanide or its salts ten times or more in excess of normally lethal doses. The concentration of rhodanese in tissue is generally proportional to that of beta-glucosidase and always functionally in excess of the latter. Rhodanese may also appear in the absence of beta-glucosidase as in the case of the brain just as beta-glucosidase may appear in conjunction with cancer or trophoblast cells in the absence of rhodanese. The high sensitivity of cerebral tissue to hypoxia would tend in the course of natural selection to provide a high rhodanese activity against adventitious HCN and to exclude any enzymatic means by which the cyanide ion could be hydrolyzed in this area. The rationale for the occurrence of a high beta-glucosidase concentration in the absence of rhodanese in the case of trophoblast is associated with the role the trophoblast plays in hemopoiesis, especially as it concerns the nitrilization of hydrocobalamin to active vitamin B12 (cyanocobalamin).

Rhodanese, beta-glucosidase, nitrilosides and thiocyanates are found throughout the phyla of the plant and animal kingdoms from bacteria to giant trees, and from protozoa to man.

THIOCYANATES IN PLANTS
Although the normally occurring nitrilosides in plants have never been known to contribute any evidence of chronic or cumulative toxicity from the nitriloside itself nor from the derivable HCN, thiocyanates occurring in plants, notably the *Cruciferae* or *Brassicae*, have been identified with goitrogenic properties among peasant populations subsisting on large quantities of such *Cruciferae* as cabbage, turnips, rutabaga, brussel sprouts, kohli rabi, cauliflower, etc. grown in iodine-deficient soil. Clovers among many other legumes and grasses are rich sources of nitriloside for grazing animals. Recently ewes grazing on nitriloside-rich clover growing in Australian soil deficient in iodine were reported as showing a high incidence of goiter which was identified as apparently arising from the thiocyanate derived from the clover nitriloside and metabolized in the presence of a severe iodine deficiency.

In soils carrying normal concentrations of iodine, no such effects have been observed in sheep or cattle despite the fact that some of these animals may ingest as much as 300 grams of nitriloside a day through dry arrow-grass, Johnson-grass, clovers, or other fodder.

It will also be recalled that Wilder Bancroft, Professor of Physical Chemistry at Cornell University, ingested 1,000 mg. of thiocyanate a day for a period of 23 years in the process of studying the cumulative properties of this chemical. He reported no untoward result from the experiment. To the contrary, he associated it with some suspected positive benefits that need not be considered at this time.

While prolonged excessive ingestion or development of thiocyanate in the presence of a severe iodine deficiency has apparently been associated with a goitrogenic effect in both human and animal populations, there has never been anything to suggest the possibility of any cumulative toxicity arising from the cyanide ion itself.

It is apparently impossible to develop cumulative toxicity to HCN in animals. The reason for this is that the biological experience with the cyanide ion in metabolism is almost as ancient and extensive as the biological experience with water, oxygen, nitrogen, salt, or the like. All can prove fatal to animals if administered in excessive quantities or in an improper way. As a result of an almost archetypical ignorance of, or superstition towards HCN engendered by observations of the swiftness of its lethality made in days when chemistry had barely emerged as a science, a powerful cultural antipathy toward cyanide developed.

Cyanide was indiscriminately and falsely classified, because of its toxic potentiality, with protoplasmic poisons utterly foreign to the biological experience of the organism. Unfortunately, this ancient misapprehension has been perpetuated among botanists, physiologists, toxicologists and even pharmacologists. And, in their culturally induced fear or antipathy toward cyanide as a poison, they have unwittingly foreclosed adequate attention to, and study of, the critically important factors in the physiology of plants and animals. An atmosphere of pure nitrogen or pure carbon dioxide is just as lethal as one of hydrogen cyanide. The major differences among these compounds possessing almost equal biological experience are those of concentrations and rates, and none are capable of producing chronic or cumulative toxicity. As we shall study in a subsequent section, sheep have received as much as 460 mg of HCN in the course of an hour without any evidence of acute toxicity and as much as 210 mg of HCN a day for two years without any evidence of cumulative toxicity or resistance or immunity of any kind to HCN. This biological experience qualitatively parallels that for water, salt, sodium chloride and compounds with similar biological experience.

Though in our early studies on the nitrilosides we attempted because of our then limited knowledge of their basic significance in terms of biological experience to ascertain some evidence of cumulative toxicity for them, we now agree with such students of the problem as Coop and Blakely that it is impossible for compounds that have, through nutrition, been a part of the biological experience of plants, animals and man and an inherent part of his physiology since his appearance, to produce any cumulative toxic effects. Whether we are dealing with the first nitriloside to be discovered, amygdalin, or with linamarin or lotaustralin, it would seem vain to expect to find from their hydrolytic products of glucose and HCN and their aglycone of benzaldehyde or benzonic acid in the case of the first, or acetone or methylethylktone, respectively, in the case of the latter, any possibility of cumulative effect. Glucose, thiocyanate, benzoic acid, and even acetone, are components normal to the metabolic pathways of the organism, which would have to be susceptible to a development of a cumulative toxicity to itself in order to sustain one to the components which comprise the organism.

If the obvious is belabored to *reductio ad absurdum,* it is because even at this late date there are apparently some unacquainted with the fact that the hydrolysis *in vivo* of a nitriloside by one or more endogenous beta-glucosidases with the production of free HCN, detoxified as thiocyanate by the enzyme rhodanese in order to protect the organism, or sometimes left undetoxified by cells or organisms lacking or deficient in rhodanese, comprises biological phenomena that were commonplace in organisms as old as man himself. As a result of a deficient rhodanese mechanism, some organisms have been destroyed by the HCN emitted by other organisms rich in beta-glucosidase and rhodanese.

Blum & Woodring *(Science,* 138:513, 1962), in a paper on "Secretion of Benzaldehyde and Hydrogen Cyanide by the Millipede *Pachydesmus crassicutis*", describe how this large millipede, whose known distribution is limited to Louisiana and southern

53

Mississippi, protects itself against its natural prey, the imported fire ant (*Solenopsis raevissima v. richteri Forel*) by secreting a mixture of benzaldehyde and hydrogen cyanide against the predator when disturbed by it. The millipede is equipped with paired glands located on eleven of the notal projections; from these glands, benzaldehyde and HCN are ejected. The water-clear secretion of *Pachydesmus* was collected by touching the dorsal surfaces of the notal projections with a small square of filter paper which rapidly absorbed the liquid discharge. This discharge was then analyzed by gas chromatography and infra red photospectroscopy. The major component was found to be benzaldehyde. HCN and glucose were also found together with a disaccharide which appears to be the sugar moiety of the nitriloside amygdalin. The millipede secretes its own beta-glucosidase, which hydrolyses the nitriloside in the notal glands to free HCN, benzaldehyde and sugar. While the millipede protects itself from the HCN through its endogenous rhodanese, this HCN is emitted against a predator relatively deficient in rhodanese.

David A. Jones, Department of Genetics, and John Parsons, Department of Pharmacology, Oxford University, in a paper on "Release of Hydrocyanic Acid from Crushed Tissues in All Stage of the Life-Cycle of Species of the Zygaeninae (Lepidoptera)" *Nature*, *193* (4810), p.52, 1962) reported that 50 crushed eggs (weight of about 50 eggs 2.6 mg - 4.0 mg) of this moth release up to 150 microgram of HCN, which HCN thus accounts for about 5 per cent of the weight of such eggs.

The foregoing examples were selected from a comprehensive body of similar data for the purpose of adumbrating the ubiquity of the biological occurrence and experience among all forms of life, not only in terms of nitriloside, but also in terms of beta-glucosidase, rhodanese, thiocyanate, and the selective susceptibility of rhodanese-deficient cells to the noxious effect of adventitious HCN. Some of the data briefly reviewed in the two papers just cited concern the occurrence of rhodanese in the parasites of the gastro-intestinal tract of animals ingesting nitriloside-rich foods. Such rhodanese is, of course, necessary as a protection against the free HCN released from the ingested nitrilosides by the beta-glucosidase produced by the intestinal flora and possibly also by the intestinal mucosa of the host.

NUTRITIONAL IMPLICATIONS

Tribes in the Karakorum of West Pakistan, the aboriginal Eskimaux, tribes of South Africa and South America living on native foods, the North American Indian in his native state, the Australian aborigines, and other native or so-called primitive peoples rely upon a diet carrying as much as 250 to 3,000 mg of nitriloside in a daily ration. All populations living close to a Neolithic level appear to be characterized dietarily by a similarly high consumption of nitriloside-rich foods.

Civilized, Westernized or Europeanized man, on the other hand, relies on a diet that probably provides an average of less than 2 mg of nitriloside a day.

It is noteworthy that no case of cancer has ever been reported among the peoples of one tribe in the Karakorums over a period of about 60 years of medical observation. For a period of at least 80 years the Eskimaux have been observed with even greater scrutiny by medical men, missionaries, teachers, traders and others for the specific purpose of attempting to discover the possible incidence of cancer among them. Despite such observations, no case of cancer has yet been reported among these two native populations while they lived on their native diet; however, in the case of the Eskimaux, a number of cancer victims have been found among those who left their original dietary habits for a Westernized diet.

The medical scrutiny by which such cancer cases were noted was no less intense than that given a large proportion of the natives not having access to modern foods.

The observations made of the Eskimaux on this subject are recorded in Vilhjalmur Stefansson's book on *"CANCER: Disease of Civilization? An Anthropological and Historical Study"* (Hill and Wang, N.Y. 1960). Philip R. White, M.D., has written an interesting preface to the book, while Rene Dubos' introductory chapter is most instructive.

The remarkable freedom primitive populations show to dental caries is, of course, a commonplace to students of anthropology. Many of the nutritional reasons for such freedom from caries among these people are not difficult to find in terms of the food that they eat, and especially of the food that they do not eat. In the similar freedom of these populations from cancer, the possible role of nutrition has been at best vague and general - as it was in the case of pellagra and the anemias prior to the discovery of the specific factor involved in the deficiency.

Major General Sir Robert McCarrison, before and during his appointment as Director of Nutrition Research in India under the Research Fund Association, treated and studied the people of Karakorum. From the perspective of 20 years of observation he reported that he had failed to find a single case of cancer among this population. Later John Clark, M.D. served in a medical mission to this population. He was properly critical of the tendency of some to romanticize the allegedly perfect health of these long-lived people. He described, as had McCarrison, a relatively high incidence of goiter among these people as well as certain skin diseases and a substantial incidence of dental caries. The nutritional basis for the high incidence of goiter among them is clear in the relative iodine deficiency of their diet. Their incidence of dental caries likewise has a clear nutritional basis. The tendency to goiter though resting on an iodine deficiency is exacerbated by the presence in their diet of an abundant quantity of nitriloside, which contributes a corresponding quantity of thiocyanate that, in the absence of adequate iodine, is goitrogenic, as we have seen in the case of human populations eating vegetables of the thiocyanate-rich *Cruciferae*, grown in areas deficient in iodine or in the case of ewes grazing on nitriloside-rich (i.e., thiocyanate-producing) clover grown in iodine deficient soil.

At any rate, John Clark, while recognizing and describing the many pathological conditions to which these people, like all others, are subject, did add that he, too, had never observed a single case of cancer among them.

While cancer may elude diagnosis in some cases, early cases ultimately become terminal cases, and when the latter involve the skin, breast, the lymphatic glands, mouth, tongue, lungs, or rectum, they do not go unrecognized even by the medically naïve - certainly not by medical observers.

DIETARY SOURCES FOR NITRILOSIDES
by Ernst T. Krebs, Jr.

KARAKORUM TRIBE

A number of reliable works have reported the general diet of the people of the Karakorum. Buckwheat peas, broad beans, lucerne, turnips, lettuce, sprouting pulse or gram, apricots with their seeds, cherries and cherry seeds, berries of various sorts - these are among the seemingly commonplace foods that comprise the bulk of the diet of these people. With the exception of lettuce and turnips, each of these plants contains some nitriloside. Turnips contain thiocyanate, a substance to which nitrilosides give rise.

Over a dozen books and articles that we have read on these people are unanimous in the report that the apricot is the major staple in their diet. In view of our work on the nitrilosides in relation to human cancer, the predominance of the apricot in the nutrition of these reportedly cancer-free people was frequently called to our attention over the years. We originally dismissed the matter on the basis of pure coincidence, especially since the meat or flesh of the apricot contains little or no nitriloside, which is concentrated in the seed that resides in the pit. The seed is the size of a small almond and may be mistaken for a shelled almond.

Finally, upon investigating the diet of these people, we found that the seed of the apricot was prized as a delicacy and that every part of the apricot was utilized. We found that the major source of fats used for cooking was the apricot seed, and that the apricot oil was so produced as inadvertently to admit a fair concentration of nitriloside or traces of cyanide into it. The apricot seed is so prized among these people that there are experts chosen among them for the purpose of testing the seeds of new apricot trees for their bitterness, since occasionally there appears strains that produce apricot seeds carrying extraordinary concentrations of nitriloside and beta-glucosidase. These trees are destroyed.

The peoples of the Karakorum share with most western scientists an ignorance of the chemistry, toxicology and physiology of the nitrilosides and nitriles. Empirically, however, they have apparently discovered the value of these factors to nutrition. They prepare a solution of HCN (prussic acid) by allowing the apricot kernel nitriloside to react, in the presence of a little water added to defatted meal, with the endogenous beta-glucosidase (emulsin) to release free HCN. The resulting solution of HCN is then maintained as a form of bitters that is added drop-wise, because of its recognized toxicity, to wines immediately before they are drunk. It is held that this solution is contributory to health and even longevity.

THE ESKIMAUX

The diet of the Karakorum is of necessity essentially a vegetable diet; that of the Eskimaux is essentially a meat diet. Superficially no two diets could probably appear more divergent; yet the Eskimaux shares with many other primitive peoples, most of whom are dominantly vegetarian, a remarkable freedom from malignant disease. On this basis we were at first inclined to dismiss the high concentration of nitrilosides in the diet of Karakorum people and others relying mainly on plant foods as simply another coincidence, contradicted by the situation among the meat-eating Eskimaux.

Upon further investigation of the Eskimaux diet we found that one berry grew abundantly in the Arctic areas and that this berry is extraordinarily rich in nitriloside. This is the salmon-berry, cloud-berry, or buffalo-berry *(Rubus spectabilis)*. It is eaten by birds, animals and men. It is also incorporated into pemmican, which is eaten during all seasons of the year. It was noted also that animals such as the caribou are important in the diet of these people. In eating the caribou, the frozen contents of the rumen or paunch are utilized as a salad and considered a delicacy. In view of this we investigated the forage upon which the caribou feeds. Among the grasses that grow in Arctic marshes, arrow-grass (*Triglochin maritima*) is very common. Studies made by the United States Department of Agriculture on the nitriloside content of arrow-grass (*Triglochin maritima*) show it to be probably richer in nitrilosides than any common grass. On a dry weight basis, one kilogram of arrow-grass was found to contain over 30,000 milligrams of nitriloside. One teaspoonful of such rumenal salad might be expected to carry 100 mg or more of nitriloside. This nitriloside is p-hydroxymandelonitrile-beta-glucoside; whereas the dominant one among the Karakorum is 1-mandelonitrile-beta-diglucoside, though both nitrilosides occur in the diet of both groups.

A quick glance at native populations in tropical areas, such as South America and South Africa, discloses a great abundance of nitriloside-containing foods. Over one-third of all plants in these areas contain nitrilosides. Cassava or manioc, sometimes described as "the bread of the tropics", is one of the most common as well as richest sources of nitriloside. As eaten by primitive populations, the bitter and nitriloside-rich manioc is preferred. People in the cities on Westernized diets favor the sweet cassava. Even in the case of these the cassava is so processed as to eliminate virtually all nitriloside or nitrile ions. The cassava eaten by those still near a Stone Age culture, on the other hand, retains a large quantity of nitriloside and nitrile ions. When these primitive and relatively cancer-free people move to the cities, the incidence of cancer among them rises, as they assume the nitriloside-free, Westernized diet. Like the rest of civilized mankind, they then show a cancer incidence of one in every three or four individuals if they live for a sufficiently long period.

RELATIVE FREEDOM OF SHEEP, GOATS, AND WILD HERBIVORES FROM CANCER

The relative freedom of wild and most domestic herbivores from cancer, as contrasted to its higher incidence among at least domesticated carnivores, has been the subject of considerable attention. The nitriloside content of much pasturage, fodder and silage is, of course, often striking. White clover *(Trifolium repens)*, alfalfa or lucerne *(Medicago sativa)*,vetch, certain millets, Johnson-grass, Sudan-grass, Arrow-grass, the various sorghums, lupines, broad beans, velvet grass, and least 80 other grasses, the leaves of *Rosacae*, berries, etc. - all are common and often rich sources of nitrilosides. The two most common of the pasture grasses, Johnson and Sudan, in many parts of the United States carry as much as 15,000 to 20,000 mgs of nitrilosides per kilogram of dry grass. A 10 kilogram ration a day is not uncommon for freely grazing animals. Such a ration would supply from 150 to 200 grams of nitriloside a day, which would upon hydrolysis yield over 10,000 mg of free hydrogen cyanide. As studies on fistulated sheep have proven, over 95 per cent of all nitrilosides ingested by herbivores in plant foods are hydrolyzed within about an hour with the release of the free HCN into the organism.

Domesticated horses, however, may be deprived of a variety of plant foods and be limited more or less to fodder completely deficient in nitriloside. In such animals the incidence of cancer appears to be reasonably high, though no formal statistics are obviously available.

WILD CARNIVORES
Carnivorous animals in their natural state treat animal food similarly to the Eskimaux of a Stone Age culture. Such animals eat the viscera, especially the rumen, and often do so before eating the muscle tissue of the animal. When carnivorous animals are domesticated as pets or maintained in zoological gardens, they often show a relatively high incidence of cancer. For example, in the great San Diego Zoo 5 bears have died in one grotto in the last 6 years. All have died from cancer of the liver. These bears were maintained on a diet almost completely free from nitrilosides. Many speculations were advanced as to the cause of their malignancy, all explanations or suggestions sharing in common a version of the virus theory of cancer. These speculations are reminiscent of those made by Sir William Osler in 1906 on the etiology of pellagra as he studied a report of about 20 per cent of the population of an asylum for the colored insane dying from pellagra during one winter. To Osler this was almost conclusive evidence for the infectious or viral or bacterial origin of pellagra.

The liver cancer, which killed the captive bears in San Diego, is suggestive of the liver cancer which kills 95 per cent of all Bantus who die from cancer in the hospitals of one area of South Africa. In their native state, liver cancer is virtually unknown among these people. When they migrate to urban areas or to the mines, their diet is changed to one consisting, for economic reasons, almost exclusively of low-grade carbohydrates completely devoid of nitrilosides. A staple of this diet is fermented milk and corn meal in a mixture known as mealie meal. When this ration was fed for a prolonged period to rats, most of the rats developed cirrhosis of the liver and the pre-cancerous changes observed in the male Bantus.

Bears in the wild state eat nitriloside-rich berries, such as choke berries, salmon berries; grasses also rich in this factor; wild fruits - apricots, peaches, apples, cherries, plums - the seeds of which are all rich in nitriloside with often the leaves and roots carrying a high concentration of the factor; and barks, roots, twigs, and flowering plants rich in nitriloside. Since bears are omnivores, they also eat game. Peter Krott, Ph.D. in his *"Bears in the Family"*, (E. P. Dutton & Co., Inc., N.Y., 1962) describes the predatory habits of the bear as follows:

"Isolated footmarks showed the shepherds where to go and it was not long before they found the remains of the sheep in the undergrowth. The body was carefully cleaned out - a butcher could not have done better. While we roasted a leg of mutton I asked the men why they did not leave the carcass in place, as the bear would surely return to finish it."

The significance of the rumenal contents of sheep in terms of nitrilosides and nitrates will become increasingly clear in the next section. The nutritional pattern in civilized man, as well as in omnivores in captivity, is reversed from what obtains in nature: the viscera is largely discarded and that which animals in the wild state treat as second rate is utilized to the exclusion of a rich source of nitrilosides.

Krott also reported the fondness of bears for whole cherries. He describes feeding two bear cubs 20 pounds of cherries. Like all the non-human primates and most primitive men, the bears eat the seeds as well as the meat of cherries.

Cancer is generally considered a chronic disease. So far no chronic or metabolic disease has ever found prophylactic or therapeutic resolution except through normally occurring accessory food factors. Certainly none has ever been known to have a viral or bacterial etiology. Pellagra, scurvy, beri-beri, rickets, the anemias, a wide range of neuropathies, etc., etc. - all have found total prophylactic and therapeutic resolution only in factors accessory to normal food. No chronic or metabolic disease has found any other resolution. It is not probable that cancer will prove the first exception.

SYSTEMATIC STUDIES OF THE NITRILOSIDE CONTENT OF VEGETABLE FOODS

by Ernst T. Krebs, Jr.

It is not practicable to attempt to list here concentrations of nitrilosides in the vegetable foods of man and all the animals. This listing is provided in our book together with a number of specimen diets or rations from the people of the Karakorum and elsewhere who live on a nitriloside-rich diet and these diets are contrasted with the inadvertently nitriloside-free diets or rations advanced by some modern nutritionists as ideal examples of the balanced diet.

Botanists, like agricultural and other experts, share our cultural antipathy toward cyanide. As a result of this antipathy, relatively slight attention has been paid to the nitriloside-containing plants, and what has been paid has been largely negative. The standard botanical technique in identifying such plants has involved a qualitative test utilizing a test tube containing a piece of filter paper moistened with a picrate solution. The suspect plant is crushed between the fingers of the botanist and then placed in the tube. A color change in the picrate paper indicates the presence of "prussic acid" [HCN]. In order for this color change to occur it is necessary, of course, that the plant contain not only the nitriloside but also the beta-glucosidase necessary to hydrolize it. Many plants contain a relatively large concentration of nitriloside with little or no beta-glucosidase, while other plants may contain only the enzyme without the nitriloside. The sweet almond is a classical example of the latter.

Agricultural experts have concerned themselves with the nitrilosides only when these have appeared in fodder and other plants in association with such high concentrations of beta-glucosidase that the plant upon being crushed immediately releases large quantities of HCN and thereby offers a threat to cattle. Such plants are labeled as "poisonous" by botanists and agricultural experts alike, and plant geneticists direct their efforts toward breeding "the cyanide" out of the plant. This, incidentally, is probably what occurred in the case of the sweet almond which, different from the bitter almond, carries only the beta-glucosidase and not the nitriloside (amygdalin).

The grasses and clovers have been virtually ignored so far as their nitriloside or nitrile content is concerned, since they seldom carry sufficient of the associated enzyme to present a toxic threat to food animals. In Australia, however, a wild fuchsia is often found in areas containing grasses very rich in the nitrilosides. The wild fuchsia is relatively low in nitriloside but rich in beta-glucosidase. Occasionally sheep or cattle grazing upon the nitriloside-rich grasses will turn to such fuschsia plants while they are in bloom and ingest the beta-glucosidase-rich foliage. As a result of this, hydrolysis of the grass nitriloside has been so accelerated that HCN has been released at a rate beyond that of the capacity of the animal to detoxify it as thiocyanate and death has quickly ensued. This situation in Australia brought about the excellent studies by Coop and Blakely of New Zealand on the physiology of nitrilosides and nitriles through the use of sheep with artificially fistulated rumen.

METABOLISM AND TOXICITY OF
CYANIDE AND NITRILOSIDES IN SHEEP
Coop and Blakely *(New Zealand Journal of Science and Technology,* 31 February 1949, page 277; ibid, 31: (3) 1; ibid, February 1950, page 45) prepared sheep with permanent rumen fistulas for the study of the production of HCN from nitrilosides and nitriloside-containing plants in the rumen. They found:

1. When HCN is introduced into the rumen, absorption is very rapid. On the average, 75% of the administered HCN is absorbed within 15 minutes.
2. Hydrolysis of nitrilosides and nitriloside-containing plants in the rumen is rapid and may be completed within 15 minutes.
3. Naturally occurring beta-glucosidase is not required because the ruminal bacteria supply this enzyme.

The rumenal bacteria supply under self-regulating conditions a source of beta-glucosidase sufficient to bring about the complete hydrolysis of nitrilosides in the ingested plant material. Regardless of the concentration of nitrilosides in the ingested plants, no toxic level of HCN is achieved because of the "self-regulating" condition under which hydrolysis is produced. Only if the nitriloside-rich vegetation is accompanied by other plant material extremely rich in beta-glucosidase is the release of HCN brought about at *a toxic rate*. Toxicity can not occur if the rate of beta-glucosidase hydrolysis is maintained at a slightly lower rate than that of rhodanese detoxification of HCN in the presence of available sulfur.

The presence of H_2S in the rumen of sheep and its rapid absorption suggests that it is probably the most important sulfur donor for HCN conversion to thiocyanate by rhodanese. While some of this conversion occurs in the rumen, probably through rumenal bacteria producing rhodanese, most of it occurs in the tissues of the animal.

Over 50 per cent of the HCN released by nitrilosides in the rumen was accounted for by thiocyanate recovered from the urine. A small quantity of free HCN is excreted by the lungs, a quantity that does not exceed 10 per cent of that produced. Additional cyanide is lost through the thiocyanates of the saliva, tears, and feces.

For all practical purposes the release of free HCN occurred at almost the same rate for nitrilosides residing in ingested plants as it did for the corresponding nitrilosides administered in the pure form.

QUANTITY OF HCN DETOXIFIED BY SHEEP

Franklin and Reid showed that normal sheep could consume the equivalent of 8 to 10mg of HCN/kg. per day as linseed meal (containing the nitriloside linamarin) without mortality.[38] In a 70 kg sheep this would be equivalent to about 700 mg of HCN. The authors found that the only way enough HCN could be administered through plant food to produce a fatal effect was to force feed the animals.

Fistulated sheep weighing 66 kg were given over a period of three hours a dose of 2.7 grams of nitriloside yielding 300 mg HCN. Coop and Blakely reported that "at no time during the experiment were even the slightest symptoms observed". A total of 568 mg HCN was given a 76 kg sheep in the course of an hour. The only symptoms the animal showed was "a general sleepiness for an hour".

---

[38] *Aust. Vet. J.*, 100: 92, 1944

WHAT IS THE 'TOXIC DOSE'
OF NITRILOSIDE OR HCN?

The toxicity of nitrilosides or the CN ion is obviously not absolute but relative to two factors:

1. The rate of hydrolysis of nitrilosides and the rate of absorption of the CN ions by the organism.
2. The rate of detoxification of the CN ion by rhodanese, in the presence of utilizable sulfur, to thiocyanate.

So long as rate (2) continues in excess of that of rate (1), toxicity from cyanide or the nitrile aspect of the nitrilosides is apparently not possible.

"Though some authors," Coop and Blakely write, *"believe that chronic cyanide poisoning is possible, it is generally recognized that, provided free HCN or cyanogenetic plants are ingested at a moderate rate throughout the course of the day, animals can tolerate amounts well in excess of the M.L.D.*[minimum lethal dose] *for a single dose. Van der Walt (Onderspoort J., 19:79,1944) failed to produce chronic poisoning in sheep even after administering 3.2 mg HCN/kg daily for two years. Worden (Vet. Records, 52. 857, 1940) showed that in rabbits repeated dosing does not produce a cumulative effect and that the animal is capable of eliminating ½ M.L.D. in 2 1/2 hours.*

On the other hand, there is no evidence that continued sublethal dosing or ingestion causes any resistance or acclimatization to HCN poisoning."

In the 70 kg sheep the dose of HCN that Van der Walt gave was 214 mg a day. This was repeated every day for two years so that the animal received a total of about 150 grains or 1/3 of a pound. No suggestion of any toxicity was found during this period and no trace of cumulative toxicity was found after two years.

To obtain the equivalent amount of nitriloside represented by the HCN, multiply the amount of HCN by the applicable nitriloside factor. For amygdalin this would be 16.92; for dhurrin, 11.51;

66

linamarin, 9.11; lotaustralin, 9.66. In addition to the free HCN component, these nitrilosides yield glucose and as an aglycone, either benzoic acid or acetone, all of which are either normal foods or normal metabolites devoid of toxicity. They account for the fact that, like free HCN itself, the nitrilosides are devoid of any chronic or cumulatively toxic properties.

Brown, Wood and Smith, in a paper on "Sodium Cyanide as a Cancer Chemotherapeutic Agent... Laboratory and Clinical Studies" *(Am. J. Obst. & Gynec., 80: 907, 1960)*, observed a similar freedom of cyanide from cumulative toxicity both in mice and human patients:

"The recovery and convalescence of these patients treated with sodium cyanide was indistinguishable from that of patients who had not received cyanide. There was no observable delayed clinical toxicity. All patients recovered promptly from the cyanide treatment and no latent or residual effects could be noted." (emphasis ours)

Though Brown, et al. reported evidence of therapeutic effects in terms of life-extension reduction in tumefaction, loss of pain, etc. in laboratory animals, in dogs, and in man, they were limited strictly by the safe peak level of 0.8 to 1.5 mg/kg of cyanide ion that can be safely presented at one time to animal tissue. Were the cyanide ion administered in such a way that a level of 0.8 mg/kg of free HCN might be approached but never exceeded - through the action of self-limiting enzyme systems on a stable source of free HCN - the period of exposure to the cyanide ion could have extended indefinitely instead of being limited to a few minutes as a result of rhodanese detoxification of CN ions not immediately replaced by other CN ions. While a 70 kg sheep was observed to be capable of receiving 506 mg of HCN over a period of four and a half hours without any suggestion of acute or chronic toxicity, a smaller dose of cyanide ion given very rapidly in a way to overwhelm the capacity of the rhodanese detoxifying system would have proven fatal. In another instance a sheep absorbed 360 mg HCN within 75 minutes whilst showing only minor symptoms. This would indicate that the capacity of the animal for HCN detoxification was about 300 mg per hour so that the sheep absorbing 506 mg of HCN within four and a half hours without any sign of toxicity fell well within the rate limits for the rhodanese system.

That parenterally administered nitrilosides are likewise subject to the self-limiting and protective capacities of the beta-glucosidase and rhodanese systems in the metabolism of free HCN is evident from numerous studies reporting the absence of parenteral toxicity for the nitriloside amygdalin. In studies conducted by our group the LD (lethal dose) for this nitriloside in rats was found to be 4.5 G./Kg. This toxicity apparently reflects that of the whole molecule rather than that of the HCN component. Such a dose would be equivalent to 315 G. of the nitriloside (intravenously administered) in a 70 g subject. This "toxicity" compares favorably with that of dextrose.

The fact that HCN is a substance with fundamental physiological significance to plant and animal organisms is indicated not only by the normal occurrence of the ion in such organisms but also by the fact that, different from such true or foreign toxins as carbon monoxide, HCN does not combine with hemoglobin unless it is first reduced to methemglobin, and even under conditions in which HCN combines with such molecules as cytochrome oxidase, this combination is highly reversible as evidenced by the fact that experimental animals even when unconscious from cyanide toxicity may be restored to consciousness (without any residual toxicity) through the administration of large quantities of rhodanese and other factors involved in the normal thiocyanate detoxification of this ion.

These facts serve to explain how cattle grazing on dry arrow-grass that may run 40,000 mg HCN per kilogram may, during a 24-hour period, ingest about 10 kilograms and safely metabolize over 400 grams of nitriloside (about a pound) in this period, which produces about 40 grams of free HCN.

Given an adequate dietary source of iodine, there is no evidence suggesting that even a goitrogenic excess of thiocyanate would develop in cattle consuming grasses as rich in nitriloside as arrow-grass. Johnson-grass and Sudan-grass are among the most common fodder grasses and a nitriloside content equal to 75 per cent that of Arrow-grass is not uncommonly found among them. That the thiocyanate produced from them presents no problem is further suggested in the fact that Professor Wilder Bancroft of Cornell ingested 1,000 mg of thiocyanate a day for 23 years and lived to the age of 88 without any sign of cumulative toxicity from the chemical. Such an amount of thiocyanate would represent the detoxification of about 450 mg of HCN a day, which would be equivalent to the quantity of HCN released from the *in vivo* hydrolysis of 7,650 mg of the amygdalin nitriloside a day. The dextrose released from such a quantity of the nitriloside would not be sufficient to raise the dextrose level from a normal 120 mg per cent in the blood to 121 mg per cent. The benzoic acid released would be equivalent to a little over a gram, which is about the quantity of benzoic acid produced through a moderate ration of certain plant foods.

It is not practicable to attempt to review here the great number of papers published during the past 164 years since L N Vauquelin first reported the identification of HCN in apricot seeds in his paper - "Expériences qui démontrent la présence de l'acide prussique tout formé dans quelque substances végétales", (*Ann. Chim.,* 45:206.1800).

From the appearance of Vauquelin's first paper in 1800 to the present, no one in the course of hundreds of papers on the subject has advanced any experimental evidence suggesting the possible cumulative toxicity of the nitrilosides such as amygdalin. Authoritative works over the world, including many editions of the *United States Dispensatory,* have properly described amygdalin as non-toxic when parenterally administered and devoid of cumulative toxicity. Certain populations have ingested in their foods up to a gram of this nitriloside a day for spans in excess of 50 years; yet such is the cultural antipathy toward the cyanides, and the misunderstanding of them therefrom resulting, that some authoritative groups have urged that the nitriloside amygdalin be studied for a period of three or four months for its possible cumulative toxicity when administered to rabbits parenterally in doses of 15 mg. kg body weight. This is despite the fact that these animals may already be ingesting plant material carrying a nitriloside content well in excess of the suggested parenteral levels.

Davison ("Synopsis of Materia Medica, Toxicology and Pharmacology", 3rd Edition, C. V. Mosby, St. Louis, 1944, p. 33) expresses the unanimous opinion of informed authority in stating: *"The glucoside amygdalin, given by injection, produces no harmful effect."*

Such common foods as lima beans may contain over a gram of nitriloside to the pound.

IN WHAT CLASSIFICATION
DO THE NITRILOSIDES FALL?
We have seen that cattle may metabolize almost a pound of nitriloside a day through their fodder, and continue to ingest large rations of nitriloside throughout the span of their life. Indeed, the better the fodder, the more nitriloside it is likely to contain.

Can the water-soluble non-toxic nitrilosides properly be described as food? Probably not in the strict sense of the word. They are certainly not drugs *per se*. They are non-toxic, and they do contribute the essential nitrile radicals to what students of physiology describe now as the "metabolic cyanide pool" in the animal organism. They foster the production of thiocyanate, are involved in the nitrilization of hydrocobalamin to active vitamin B12 or cyanocobalamin, and they exert a physiological effect that, when sufficient, is reflected in a hypotensive reaction. They do not depress any vital function such as hemopoiesis. To the contrary, their CN ion has been repeatedly reported as raising both the red cell count and the total hemoglobin in animals and humans given small quantities of cyanides or various quantities of the nitrilosides.

Since the nitrilosides are neither food nor drug, they may be considered as accessory food factors. *Another term for water-soluble, non-toxic accessory food factors is vitamin.*

THERAPEUTIC IMPLICATIONS
We have glanced briefly at populations almost or entirely free from cancer under dietary conditions native to them. One such population was seen to be almost exclusively vegetarian; the other, almost exclusively meat-eating. These populations shared in common a high consumption of nitrilosides. We live in a

civilization in which one out of every 3 or 4 of us will develop cancer. Our population is characterized by a dietary pattern almost devoid of nitrilosides.

We have seen animals that, in their native state, are almost devoid of cancer. Observing these animals in captivity, we see an alarming increase in the incidence of cancer in them. These animals, whether they be the 5 bears in the San Diego Zoo that died from cancer over the past six years, or cats and dogs in our household, share one common dietary experience: an almost total deficiency in nitrilosides in contrast to the abundance of this factor in their natural diet. To these generalizations on the increased incidence of cancer in domestic animals we find a remarkable exception in sheep and cattle. But when we examine their ration, we find it extremely rich as a rule in the nitrilosides. An exception sometimes is found to this in work horses. Here we find the incidence of cancer strangely elevated. Such animals are usually maintained on a nitriloside-free ration of oats and timothy hay and the like.

We frequently observe cats and dogs that, under domestication, are provided with a variety of rich foods seek out a garden or a weed patch and commence to eat Johnson-grass, even certain species of crab-grass, and other grasses. These grasses have in common a high nitriloside content. In the wild state we see even the omnivorous bear eat first the nitriloside- and nitrile-filled rumen of sheep while leaving the mutton legs and the remainder of the carcass for a period of hunger.

Among the poor of rural Turkey the incidence of cancer is substantially lower than in the West. Professor Sayre, in the May 1960 issue of the *New England Journal of Medicine,* published a paper on "Health Hazards, Cyanide Poisoning from Apricot Seeds among Children in Central Turkey". The children involved had mistaken the wild apricot for the domestic variety. The wild variety carries seeds containing 2,000 mg of HCN per Kg., equivalent to about 35 grams of the nitriloside. The nitriloside existing in the presence of a rich concentration of beta-glucosidase in these seeds renders them toxic. But adults and children in Central Turkey prize these seeds as a delicacy, and parents believing they are "good for the health" do not dissuade their children from eating them.

In the June 1964 issue of *Gourmet Magazine*, there appeared a letter explaining that since China does not have a true almond, the nut of the apricot is used in its place. This letter caused a physician's wife to write in alarm warning the Editor against the food use of apricot kernels. The Editor for a time shared her alarm until he consulted with the U.S. Food and Drug Administration (FDA), the Poisons Control Center of New York City Department of Public Health, and others. The consensus was that the seeds were safe for human consumption because the quantities used are usually small and cooking provides an additional safeguard (through destroying the beta-glucosidase).

All this is despite the fact that all the sub-human primates that eat apricots, plums, cherries, peaches, apples, and the like also eat the seeds. All the primates fed these fruits in zoos are seen tediously to extract and eat the seeds from pits as resistant even as the apricot. All people of the Stone Age culture, so far as we have been able to ascertain, eat the seeds of all fruits - almost all of which are extremely rich in nitrilosides.

ORIGINAL STUDIES
by Ernst T. Krebs, Jr.

Over a decade ago, clinical investigation of then empirical extracts from apricot kernels *(prunus armeniaca)* was commenced because of evidence of some anti-neoplastic activity in animals. In humans this extract proved to be palliative in human cancer. Further study showed the responsible factor to be the nitriloside amygdalin. This nitriloside (Laetrile) was then chosen as the subject for systematic clinical investigation after its lack of immediate or cumulative toxicity was demonstrated on experimental animals.

The doses of the nitriloside standardized for human use range from about 12.5 mg/kg to 37.5 mg/kg of the nitriloside. These doses supply from 0.8 mg/kg of the HCN ion. Doses as high as 20 grams or more intravenously have been shown to be without toxic effect in healthy human subjects, though a mildly hypotensive effect is produced through the thiocyanate engendered by such large doses. It appears that the 0.8 mg/kg (equivalent to a dose of 1.0 gram of the nitriloside in a 70 kg patient) is generally optimal.

Brown, Wood and Smith in their studies on sodium cyanide in mice bearing Sarcoma 180 found experimentally that 0.8 mg./kg of the CN ion was the optimal dose in contributing a life-extension of as high as 70 per cent to not only these mice but to another strain bearing Ehrlich's ascites cell tumors. Not only did such doses lack cumulative toxicity; but the controls not receiving the cyanide obviously experienced a 70 per cent shorter lifespan.

Brown et al. were unaware of any work on nitriloside during the period they made their studies; yet the optimal dosage of the nitrile ion they arrived at from studies on cancer animals is identical to the optimal dose determined for clinical use for nitriloside (Laetrile) by many clinical investigators working over the course of a decade while gradually scaling their original doses of 50mg of the nitriloside to the present dose of 1,000 mg and altering the route of administration from intramuscular one to an intravenous one. Brown et al observed:

"Because the action of... cyanide is almost instantaneous and since normal tissues and cells are capable of recovering from its noxious effects, it could be anticipated here that there would be no cumulative or latent complications in the bone marrow, the gastrointestinal tract, or the renal apparatus."

Clinical experience with approximately 100,000 parenteral doses of nitriloside in man over a decade of study have sustained Brown's original findings on the non-toxicity of the CN ion administered within the capacity of the rhodanese system. Administration of the ion in the form of nitriloside of course provides an optimal concentration of the ion in a safe and self-limiting fashion - self-limitation being the characteristic of the action of accessory food factors.

Maxwell and Bischoff in 1933, in studying the possible cumulative effect of HCN in mice, reported:

"After twenty-one days of exposure to HCN, the red blood cell count and the hemoglobin rose in the mice 12 to 15 per cent, and in the rats, 20 to 25 per cent." [39]

Their experience has been confirmed repeatedly by clinicians studying the action of Laetrile (nitriloside) in advanced cases of human cancer where the nitriloside-derived HCN has produced a substantial stimulation in hemopoiesis even in some terminal patients.

In 1935, Isabella Perry of the Department of Pathology, University of California Medical School, reported on the study of "The Effects of Prolonged Cyanide Treatment on the Body and Tumor Growth in Rate" *(American Journal of Cancer,* 25:592). Reporting the action of prolonged inhalation of cyanide fumes in young tumor-bearing rats, she wrote:

"...Retards the growth of Jensen sarcoma implants. A considerable percentage of the animals so treated showed complete regression of the tumor. Both regressing and growing tumors in treated

---

[39] *J. Pharmacol. & Exper. Therap.*, 49:270

animals had little capacity for transplantation... The dose was given on strips of blotter paper...It seems that the range of the effective dose is limited and too close to the lethal dose to be practical."

The administration of CN ion through non-toxic nitrilosides eliminates the limitation. Perry observed that:

"In the treated animals the tumors grew slowly and necrosed early. Ten days after the inoculation, the tumors in 9 treated rats averaged 0.5 cm in diameter, while the 8 control rats had tumors averaging 2.2 cm in diameter. On the twenty-fifth day after the tumors had been inoculated and fifteen days after the cyanide treatment was discontinued, 5 treated survivors had <u>tumors</u> averaging 2.5 cm in diameter, while the tumors in the control animals averaged 8 cm in diameter."

Of the control rats bearing Jensen sarcoma, 8 had died and only one was surviving on the 34th day after inoculation. By the 105th day, 6 treated rats that had received the same implantation were still alive and showed extensive tumor regression. Such residues which remained were untransplantable. Thus treated by the inhalation of HCN gas, with all its attendant dangers, rats bearing Jensen sarcoma transplanted often showed not only complete tumor regression but an average life extension in excess of 300 per cent.

These observations have been substantiated clinically with the nitriloside-derived CN ion of Laetrile and without any evidence of toxicity and no side-effect except the increase in red blood cell count and hemoglobin first observed in 1933 by Maxwell & Bischoff in mice receiving cyanide ions.

Clinical investigation of parenteral nitriloside (Laetrile) at four universities' medical schools over the past decade have confirmed the animal studies reporting a specific chemotherapeutic effect of the CN ion in cancer. Professor M. D. Navarro of the University of St. Thomas Medical School has observed such effects for Laetrile (nitriloside) over a period of twelve years.

One gram of Laetrile (nitriloside) treated with beta-glucosidase derived from the tissues of experimental animals (with or without cancer) supplies 56 mg of HCN. This HCN may be administered through inhalation to cancer animals as in the case of Perry's studies. It may be neutralized with NaOH, to form sodium cyanide and then so administered as in the case of the work by Brown et al who found that 0.8 mg/kg of the cyanide ion provided a 70 per cent life extension in experimental animals and an apparently complete regression in spontaneous cancer in dogs as well as substantial palliation in some human cases. Under experimental conditions, Laetrile (nitriloside) has been hydrolyzed by a few drops of beta-glucosidase to a solution of free HCN, sugar and benzaldehyde. In this state the material, of course, becomes as toxic as the materials used by Brown et al, Perry, Maxwell & Bischoff and others and provides the same action as such.

FOCAL ACTION OF LAETRILE (NITRILOSIDE)
by Ernst T. Krebs, Jr.

Some of the findings reporting a selective action for CN on a diversity of malignant tumors in various animals have been briefly reviewed. In all these cases the administration of the CN ion was presented to the tissues of the organism diffusely and at an uniform concentration whether through injection of a cyanide salt or through inhalation. We have pointed out that, by the prior hydrolysis of Laetrile (nitriloside) *in vitro*, the injection of the hydrolyzed material (before and after neutralization with NaOH) or its administration through the vaporization of HCN would present the organism with precisely the same chemicals in the same quantities as in the described experiments.

When the nitriloside however is parenterally administered, as such it enters the bloodstream as an intact molecule. Malignant lesions are focally characterized by an especially high and selective concentration of beta-glucosidase and beta-glucuronidase. An extensive literature describes the high focal concentration of beta-glucuronidase that characterizes most malignant lesions. This concentration is often in excess of 300 times that of the contiguous somatic tissues. There is also a substantial literature describing the deficiency of the definitively malignant cell in rhodanese. The occurrence of beta-glucuronidase appears to be paralleled by an equal concentration of beta-glucosidase. Both enzymes are described generically as *beta-glucosidases*. Synthetic glucuronosidic nitrilosides (Laetrile) have been synthesized to exploit the beta-glucuronidase system in the same manner in which the natural nitrilosides are used against the beta-glucosidase system at the malignant lesion. In comparative studies, it has been found that both the natural and synthetic nitrilosides are active against their respective enzyme systems. The simple natural nitriloside however has been chosen for our routine investigation at this time.

This nitriloside is selectively hydrolyzed at the malignant lesion by the beta-glucosidase in the rhodanese-deficient lesion. In this way the CN ion is brought to the malignant cell in a highly concentrated and selective manner. It is true that there are a number of normal tissues in the body that carry both beta-glucosidase and beta-glucuronidase, but they also carry a countervailing concentration of rhodanese, which completely protects such normal somatic tissue from the action of any cyanide ion that the beta-glucosidase or beta-glucuronidase component of the tissue causes to be released from the hydrolyzed nitriloside. In each instance the rhodanese capacity in such tissues is proportional to, though in excess of, the beta-glucosidase capacity. This prevents the diffusion of the hydrolyzed CN and accounts for the fact that Laetrile (nitriloside) is completely non-toxic to somatic or non-malignant tissue, while being extremely and selectively toxic to the specific malignant cells that provide a situation in which nitriloside is hydrolyzed at a rapid rate in the absence of an adequate rhodanese system. While the studies by Berry, Brown et al., Maxwell and Bischoff have shown in experimental animals, in domestic pets bearing spontaneous cancers, and in man that the malignant cell is selectively susceptible to cyanide ions diffusely and uniformly distributed among all body cells, the clinical work on Laetrile (nitriloside), as well as the early animal work, has shown that the selective susceptibility of the cancer cell to HCN may further be exploited through the phenomenon of selective lysis at the malignant lesion.

The equivalency of the derivable HCN of nitriloside to that of NaCN and HCN used by Brown et al and Perry respectively has been stressed almost to an absurdity for the purpose of emphasizing that in non-toxic, water-soluble, accessory food factors normal to the adequate diet of the higher animals and man, there exists a component that will bring about the total regression of a variety of cancers in experimental animals, reduce the size of other malignant lesions 8-fold or more, prevent by 10-fold or more the rate of malignant growth as compared to that seen in control animals bearing the same tumor, and render the treated tumors insusceptible to transplantation and the treated animals resistant to the implantation of cancer, as compared to controls showing full transplantability as well as full receptivity to malignant transplants.

The effect of rendering the malignant tumor untransplantable and rendering the treated animal insusceptible to the transplantation of a malignant tumor, are expressive of *prophylactic effects*. Like all other non-toxic, water-soluble, accessory food factors that have been identified as specific in a given chronic or metabolic disease, the specificity of nitriloside is also accompanied by a specific prophylactic effect.

To emphasize again the equivalency of the cyanide ion in nitriloside as compared to the free ion or its salt, we may point out that many nitriloside-rich food plants need merely to be mashed in their native state and allowed to stand awhile in their own fluid to cause them to surrender the free HCN that can duplicate what has already been achieved by this ion in experimental animals bearing transplanted or spontaneous cancer. This is the non-toxic, water-soluble accessory food factor that is as important to adequate nutrition as ascorbic acid, thiamine, riboflavin and similar non-toxic, water-soluble accessory food factors that appear in plants in a lower concentration, as a rule, than does nitriloside.

UNIFORMITY OF EFFECT
It will be noted that the CN ion did not produce a total regression of all tumors in all animals. It brought about a total regression of a good variety of tumors in four or more species of animals. It also accounted for an average life-extension of 70 per cent in one group and extension as high as 300 per cent in another group. Of all achievements, failure is the most facile to attain. There have been several investigators who sought to prove that Laetrile (nitriloside) had no action in experimental animals bearing cancers. The longest study done involved less than six weeks and transplanted Jensen sarcoma. The investigator failed to achieve "objective results" in this period, and discounted the soundness of the experiment on the declared grounds that animal tissue contained no means to hydrolyze nitriloside to free HCN - that animal tissue does not contain beta-glucosidase. Such incompetence of a presumably honest nature has characterized many of the mistaken notions that experimental demonstration is gradually eliminating from this area.

CLINICAL STUDIES
We have written nothing about the very extensive and very successful clinical investigation of nitriloside (Laetrile) that has been conducted by a number of highly competent workers over the world. Without exception, all of these men have reported one

degree of success or another in advanced or terminal cases. No one who has actually used and studied the material has failed to report positive results, though many who have neither used nor studied the material have criticized it. Such critics have described the provable positive results, and even recoveries that have followed the use of nitriloside (Laetrile) in late or terminal cancer patients as an expression of "the delayed therapeutic effects of prior radiation, surgery or other chemotherapy". Since only advanced cases in which such measures have already failed have so far been given Laetrile (nitriloside), all such cases are theoretically subject to the critical explanation described. One clinician has pointed out that if nitriloside itself does not directly produce the results that usually follow its application, it does greatly increase the percentage of "delayed therapeutic effects" that follow seemingly unsuccessful prior measures. One can but anticipate that, when the nitrilosides are finally used in the treatment of those cancers previously untreated by other methods, the incidence of spontaneous remissions will be found by such critics to have increased beyond reasonable statistical expectations.

THE UNITARIAN OR TROPHOBLASTIC THESIS
OF CANCER[40]

(reprinted from the *Medical Record* for July 1950)

BY ERNST T. KREBS, JR.
ERNST T. KREBS, SR.[41]
and
HOWARD H. BEARD[42]

[40] We wish to acknowledge the helpful suggestions and criticisms on the trophoblastic thesis from Clifford L. Bartlett, M.D., Pasadena, California; John Bodman M.D., London, England; and Arthur Harris, M.D., North Hollywood, California.
[41] John Beard Memorial Foundation, 642, Capp Street, San Francisco, California.
[42] Cancer Clinic, Holy Cross Hospital, Chicago, Illinois.

It is veritably impossible to find, among the hundreds of valid experimental contributions to our knowledge of cancer made during the past half century, an experimentally established datum that would contravert the thesis of the basic biological uniformity characterizing all exhibitions of cancer.

THE CRITERIA OF UNIFORMITY

To the experimentalist who does not overtly accept a unitarian thesis of cancer, such a thesis is still implicit in the commonplace facts of his science. The classic experiments of Warburg on the respiratory pattern of cancers of various species and tissue origins reveal a high uniformity from tumor to tumor.[43] Correlatively, the Cori's find the lactic acid and sugar content of the various exhibitions of cancer to be highly uniform.[44] Williams and his co-workers report a pronounced degree of uniformity in the concentration of eight B vitamins in a great variety of animal and human tumors, regardless of the tissue of their origin or the manner of their induction.[45] Robertson makes similar observations for vitamin C.[46] The addition of various substrates to malignant tumors of various types yields highly uniform respiratory responses.[47] Shack describes an almost complete uniformity in cytochrome oxidase content in a number of mouse tumors.[48] Greenstein finds that the presence of any exhibition of cancer uniformly results in a depression of the liver catalase.[49] [50] Maver and Barrett describe substantial evidence for an immunological

---

[43] Warburg, O.: "Stoflwechsel d. Tumore", Springer, Berlin, 1926. Engl. Edn., "The Metabolism of Tumors", tr. F. Dickens, London, 1930

[44] Cori, C. F. and Cori, C. J.: *J. Biol. Chem.*, 64,1.:11, 1925

[45] Williams, R. J.: Symposium on Cancer, A. A. A. S. Research Conference on Cancer, ed. F. R. Moulton, Am. Assoc. Advancement of Science, Washington, D.C,. 1945, p. 253

[46] Robertson, W. V.: *J. Natl. Cancer Inst.* 4:321, 1943

[47] Kidd, J. G.; Winzler, R. J. and Burk, D.: *Cancer Research* 4.547, 1944

[48] Shack, J.: *J. Natl. Cancer Inst.* 3:389, 1943

[49] Greenstein, J. P.: Symposium on Cancer, A. A. A. S. Research Conference on Cancer, ed. F. R. Moulton, Am. Assoc. Advancement of Science, Washington, D. C., 1945, p.192

[50] Greenstein, J. P., Jenrette, W. V. and White, J.: *J. Natl. Cancer Inst.* 2:283, 1941

uniformity among malignant tumors.[51] Greenstein reports an impressive degree of uniformity in enzyme concentration among malignant tissues, regardless of their means of induction, tissue of origin or species of origin.[52] Others describe a uniformly low content of such aerobic catealytic systems as cytochrome, succinic, and d-amino acid oxidases, cytochrome-c, catalase and flavin.[53] [54] [55] [56] [57] [58] [59]

Further phenomena of uniformity are observed in the elevated water and cholesterol of the malignant tumors as well as other primitive tissues. [60] [61] The induction by a single steroid carcinogen, such as methylcholanthrene, of malignant exhibitions as diverse as leukemia and malignant melanoma, attests to a basically uniform etiology. The uniformity of various exhibitions of cancer in respiratory properties, lactic acid production, vitamin content, enzyme content, action on a given substrate, effect on liver catalase, cytochrome oxidase content, immunological properties, and many other characteristics is correlative to a uniformity of malignant tumors in the ability to metastasize, in their amenability to heterotransplantability, and in their autonomy, invasiveness and erosiveness.[62] [63] Indeed, there is no known basic property unique to any single exhibition of cancer - the only variation being a morphological one partially conditioned by admixed benign or somatic components.

[51] Maver, M. E. and Barrett, M. K.: *J. Natl. Cancer Inst.* 4:65, 1943

[52] Greenstein, J. P.: *Biochemistry of Cancer*, Academic Press, New York, 1947

[53] Schneider, W. C. and Potter, V.R. *Cancer Research* 3:353, 1943

[54] Robertson, W. Y.B. and Kahler, H.: *J. Natl. Cancer Inst.* 2:595, 1942

[55] Du Bois, K.P. and Potter, V.R.: *Cancer Research* 2:290, 1942

[56] Greenstein, J. P., Edwards, J. E., Andervont, H. B. and White, J.: *J. Natl. Cancer Inst.* 3:7, 1942

[57] Rosenthal, O. and Drabkin, D. L.: *J. Biol. Chem.* 150: 131, 1943

[58] Greenstein, J. P., Werne, J., Eschenbrenner, A. B. and Leuthardt, F. M.: *J. Natl. Cancer Inst.* 5:55, 1944

[59] Okuneff, N. and Nasarbekowa, *Ztsch, f.Krebforsch*, 41:28, 1934

[60] Needham, J.: *Chemical Embryology*, Cambridge, 1931, p. 884, 1948

[61] Burgheim, F. and Joel, W.: *Klin. Wchnschr.* 8:828, 1929.9 10:397, 1931

[62] Greene, H. S. N.: *Yale J. Biol. and Med.* 18:239, 1946

[63] Greene, H. S. N., Lund, P. K., *Cancer Research* 4:352, 1944

The degree in the uniformity of the factors described increases with the increasing malignancy with which the tumor is exhibited. Thus with an increasing degree of malignancy, all malignant exhibitions converge toward a common tissue type. For this reason the cells of the most malignant of all exhibitions of cancer should epitomize the properties of the malignant component in all other exhibitions of cancer. That this is the case, we shall observe in the pages that follow.

We have glanced briefly at data that are commonplace to cancer research. The logical consequences of these data have, however, seldom been examined. Since the phenomenon of cancer is truly a unitarian one, then, of logical necessity, the variations in the biological malignancy of different exhibitions of cancer must be a function of *the concentration of a cell of an intrinsically uniform malignancy.*

POSITION OF THE CANCER CELL IN THE LIFE-CYCLE

In accounting for the nature and origin of the single cell type comprising the constant malignant component in the varying morphological exhibitions of cancer, we find one of two alternatives open. The definitively malignant cell either has its normal counterpart in the life-cycle or the malignant cell is without a normal, cellular counterpart and, therefore, arises as a spontaneous generation. Since spontaneous generation is an untenable postulate, the only alternative is that the malignant cell has its counterpart in the life-cycle. The question then arises whether this counterpart is a relatively developed cell or the most primitive cell in the life-cycle. Since the primitivity of the cancer cell is a commonplace, in looking for its cellular counterpart in the life-cycle, we turn to the most primitive cell in this cycle. This is the trophoblast cell. Then as a logical corollary of the unitarian thesis, we should find the trophoblast cell as the constant malignant component in all exhibitions of cancer: the malignancy of the cancer varying directly with its concentration of trophoblast cells and inversely with its concentration of somatic cells.

If the unitarian thesis is valid, then the most malignant exhibition of cancer possible should be comprised almost completely of *frank* trophoblast cells; and, in being so comprised, should epitomize the cellular and other phenomena shared by exhibitions of a lesser malignancy. The most highly malignant exhibitions of cancer known are the chorionepitheliomas comprised of frank *trophoblast cells,* cytologically early, endocrinologically and otherwise indistinguishable from normal pregnancy trophoblast cells. If cancer is an unitarian phenomenon whose malignancy is a function of the concentration of trophoblast cells within a given tissue, then the greater the concentration of such cells within a tissue, the higher the malignancy of the tissue and the more profound its cytological deviation from the cytology normal to the tissue. If the unitarian thesis is valid, then the single exception to this generalization would comprise the most malignant of all exhibitions of cancer: that involving the pathologic exhibition of the normally or "physiologically" malignant pregnancy trophoblast. It is, therefore, most significant that when pregnancy trophoblast is malignantly exhibited as primary uterine chorionepithelioma, there is no *ascertainable cytological, endocrinological or other intrinsic change whatever from the normal trophoblast cell.* As Boyd has phrased it, "microscopically the chorionepithelioma is an exaggeration of the condition normally found in pregnancy."[64] All other tumors represent an attenuation of the condition of their normal tissue of origin.

PROPERTIES OF THE TROPHOBLAST CELL

But if cancer is, as a unitarian phenomenon, trophoblastic then we should expect to find occasionally in the male - where trophoblast never normally exists - at least some cases in which the failure in somatic resistance to the definitive malignant cell (trophoblast cell) is so complete that the trophoblast is frankly exhibited as such in the fiercely malignant testicular or primary extra-genital chorionepitheliomas.[65] [66] [67] [68] [69] The chorionepitheliomas are unquestionably the most malignant tumors in either sex, and the degree of their malignancy is routinely determined by measuring

---

[64] Boyd, W.: *Textbook of Pathology*, Lea & Febiger, ed. 4th, Philadelphia, 1943

[65] Truc, E. and Guibert, H. L.: *Bull Assoc. Cancer* 26:319, 1937

[66] McDonald, S.: *Am. J. Cancer* 24:1, 1938

[67] Hellwig, A. C.: *Urol. and Cutan. Rev.* 48:53, 1944

[68] Gill, A. J., Caldwell, G. T. and Goforth J. L.: *Am. J. Med. Sci.* 210:745, 1945

[69] Petillo, D.: *Urol. and Cutan. Rev.* 48:53, 1944

the gonadotrophin [hCG hormone] their trophoblast cells excrete.[70]
[71] [72] [73]

If the trophoblast cell, presented outside the normal canalization or checks of pregnancy, is truly the cancer cell, then it must be impossible for the trophoblast cell or its hormone - "chorionic" gonadotrophin - ever to be found in the male or, aside from the canalization of normal pregnancy, in the female except in a malignant fashion. *Neither the trophoblast cell nor its hormone has ever been so found except as cancer.* And whenever the trophoblast cell or its hormone has been found in the male or the non-pregnant female, the associated malignancy is observed to vary directly with the urinary excretion of trophoblast cell-produced gonadotrophin.

Even a superficial examination of the trophoblast cell indicates that it possesses such properties of the cancer cell as invasiveness, erosiveness, autonomy, and ability to metastasize throughout the organs of the host."[74] [75] Indeed, though normally canalized to physiological ends, the pregnancy trophoblast, in carrying the conceptus from anatomically outside of the maternal host to implantation within the uterine wall, must behave in a profoundly malignant fashion. No malignant cell invades any tissue any more rapidly and completely than the pregnancy trophoblast does the human uterus in the first few weeks of gestation.

If the trophoblast cell, then, is *intrinsically* malignant, this malignancy should become especially apparent when the trophoblast is removed from the normal extrinsic checks and controls surrounding it in its normal canalization of pregnancy. Maximov is among those who have observed normal pregnancy trophoblast in tissue culture *pari passu* non-trophoblast.[76] He

---

[70] Francis, R. S.: *Brit. J. Surg.* 33:173, 1945

[71] Fortner, H. C. and Owen, S. E.: *Am. J. Cancer* 25:89, 1935

[72] *Editorial, Am. Int. Med.* 5, 1931

[73] hCG is the hormone pregnancy tests seek in order to render a positive result.

[74] Ewing, J.: *Neoplastic Diseases*, Saunders, Philadelphia, 1940.

[75] Adami, J. C.: *Medical Contributions to the Study of Evolution*, Macmillan, New York, 1918, p. 286

[76] Maximov, A.: Carnegie Contrib. *Embryol.* 16:47, 1924

describes as follows a tissue culture preparation of a normal rabbit embryo *plus* the contiguous trophoblast:

"From the very first moment of their formation in vitro, the trophoblastic elements, whose function under normal conditions is to destroy, resorb, and penetrate into the uterine mucosa, attack the growing embryonic tissues. They glide between the cells through the intercellular spaces, along blood vessels, gnaw large holes in epithelia sheet... Wherever they appear they dissolve, destroy and resorb everything surrounding them. <u>The picture sometimes bears a striking resemblance to chorionepithelioma malignum</u>. As in vitro, there is no maternal tissue, the destructive tendencies of the trophoblast are directed toward the next and only available - the embryonic tissue itself. This is rapidly destroyed and totally used up for the nutrition and growth of the trophoblast." [emphasis ours]

Maximov's description of the nutritive utilization by the trophoblast of somatic or embryonic tissue *in vitro* bears a striking parallelism to the following observation of Greenstein[77] on the nutritive behavior of the cancer cell:

"It is, indeed, astonishing that a tumor can thus attach itself to an organism already running downhill in negative nitrogen balance and subsequently grow at the host's further expense."

Parasitization is eloquently clear in the description given by Maximov and it is implicit in Greenstein's observation. Normal pregnancy trophoblast represents, of course, a parasitization of cells of one genetic constitution by those of another. If cancer is a unitarian, and thereby a trophoblastic phenomenon, its parasitic behavior is very easy to understand.

Were pregnancy trophoblast *in vivo* or *in situ* to lack the humorally mediated checking influences that are lacking *in vitro,* then such tissue would expectedly behave as it does *in vitro* and be exhibited

---

[77] Greenstein, J. P.: *Biochemistry of Cancer*, Academic Press, New York, 1947, p.151

in the fiercely malignant fashion of primary uterine chorionepithelioma.

Rather than pause here to review in further detail the points of identity between the cancer cell and the trophoblast cell, of which the senior author in a review of over 17,000 papers has been able to catalogue 43, let it suffice to say that we have been unable to find a single point of dissimilarity between the cancer cell and the pregnancy trophoblast cell. The points of identity, of course, are those shared exclusively by the cancer cell and the trophoblast cell and not shared by any somatic cell.

THE CELL OF ORIGIN AND THE
MEANS OF ITS DIFFERENTIATION

If cancer is a truly unitarian phenomenon, then its cellular origin as well as its cellular nature are exemplified in the origin and nature of the most malignant exhibition of cancer - primary uterine chorionepithelioma.

Pregnancy trophoblast arises through the *differentiation* by meiosis of a diploid totipotent [stem] cell in response to *organizer stimuli* (afforded through the sex steroids). The meiosis of the diploid totipotent cell results in a haploid gametogenous cell, whose only alternative to death is division (sexually or parthenogenetically induced) with the consequent production of trophoblast. The only cell from which the most primitive cell in the life-cycle, the trophoblast cell, can arise is the most undifferentiated or most potent cell in the life-cycle: the diploid totipotent [stem] cell. It is this cell alone that is competent for meiosis. In fact, aside from the explanation of spontaneous generation, only two alternatives exist for the origin of the malignant cell. Like all other growth phenomena, it may arise as the result of the differentiation of an undifferentiated cell in response to organizer stimuli; alternatively, it may be ascribed to the ontogenetic "reversion" of normal cells to a primitive state. Even though the very notion of such reversion is a thermodynamic fantasy inadmissible by modern biology, if a normal cell *could* revert, the most primitive cell in the life-cycle toward which such reversion could occur is still the trophoblast cell. Hence, aside from the errors of spontaneous generation or cellular reversion, *only the phenomena of cellular differentiation are tenable in accounting for the origin of the cancer cell - though the signals to such differentiation may, of course, be diversely mediated.*

It is thus a simple embryological fact that the malignant component of the most malignant of all exhibitions of cancer - primary uterine chorionepithelioma - represents the unchecked growth of normal trophoblast that has arisen through the differentiation of a diploid totipotent [stem] cell, by reduction division, and the division of the consequent haploid gametogenous cell to produce trophoblast. We have seen the proof of this in the fiercely malignant behavior of rabbit trophoblast removed from the checking influence of the maternal host and placed in tissue culture. This trophoblast, of course, came into being through processes normal to the production of all trophoblast in normal gestation. This is true also of the trophoblast of primary uterine chorionepithelioma.

It is necessary that we emphasize here the fact that our description of the origin of *any* trophoblast cells is merely a recapitulation of commonplace, universally accepted embryological data. We must not permit terminology to obscure this fact. Let us add that it has been experimentally established that in mammals the haploid gametogenous cell in either the male or the female may be non-sexually activated into division with the consequent and inevitable production of trophoblast.

Because the trophoblast cell of primary testicular chorionepithelioma is indistinguishable from that of the normal pregnancy trophoblast cell[78] [79] [80] or a trophoblast cell of primary uterine chorionepithelioma,[81] [82] the general consensus in pathology that chorionepitheliomas arise from the division of a gametogenous cell (non-sexually activated), derived through the normal meiosis of a diploid totipotent [stem] cell, is biologically and logically sound.

---

[78] Ross, J.M.: *J. Path. and Bact.* 35:563, 1932

[79] Twombly, G.H.: in a symposium on Endocrinology of Neoplastic Diseases, Oxford Univ. Press, New York, 1947, p.228 ff.

[80] Gallens, J.: *J. de sc. Méd. De Lille* 53:129, 1935

[81] Entwhistle, R.M. and Hepp, J.A.: *J.A.M.A*, 104:395, 1935

[82] Solcard, P., Le Chinton, F., Perves, J., Berge, C. and Penaneach, J: *Bull. du cancer* 25:801, 1936

It is likewise generally recognized that *primary extra-genital* chorionepitheliomas occurring in both sexes represent trophoblast that shares a common cellular origin with all other trophoblast: an origin from an haploid gametogenous cell (through fertilization or non-sexually) that has arisen through the meiosis of a diploid totipotent cell. This principle is congruent with the axiom that cells which are alike arise from pre-existing cells that are alike.

INDEX OF MALIGNANCY

If cancer is a unitarian phenomenon in which all morphological exhibitions share, in varying degrees, the known malignant component of the chorionepitheliomas, then it follows:

1. that the malignancy of a growth will vary directly with its concentration of trophoblast cells and inversely with its concentration of body or somatic cells; and
2. the trophoblast cells comprising a malignant lesion must possess the capacity for being morphologically masked or obscured by the tissue in which they primarily occur or to which they metastasize.

Testicular chorionepitheliomas afford an interesting vantage point for the examination of these possibilities. In screening over 900 testicular cancers in the Army Institute of Pathology, Friedman and Moore (1946) reported, in part, as follows:

"Nearly twice as many metastases which exhibited chorionepitheliomatous structures arose from primary tumors containing no chorionepithelioma as from pure chorionepitheliomasa or neoplasms containing focal chorionepithelioma. While only 0.4 per cent of the primary testicular tumors were pure chorionepitheliomas and 6.4 per cent showed focal chorionepitheliomatous tissue, 27 per cent of all metastases which terminated fatally contained chorionepitheliomatous elements."[83] (emphasis ours)

Thus, not only may the trophoblast, when frankly exhibited as such in the primary site, metastasize to be morphologically masked in

---

[83] Friedman, N.B. and Moore, R.A.: *Military Surgeon* 99:573, 1946

the secondary site, but the primary trophoblast itself may be morphologically masked by the soma and be frankly exhibited only when metastases occur into tissues of relatively lower reactivity in which the trophoblast is not morphologically masked but is frankly exhibited as such. The masking of the trophoblast by the reactivity of the somatic cells is a measure of the resistance of the host: the degree to which such somatic resistance against the ectopic trophoblast fails determines the malignancy with which the trophoblast is exhibited. Thus, the greater the incidence of a chorionepitheliomatous exhibition (trophoblast) in the metastases, the greater the degree of malignancy.

COMPETENT CELL AND ORGANIZER

The origin of every new cell is the result of the apposition of a competent cell and an organizer stimulus. All new cells arise as the result of cellular differentiation, which is a process by which a new cell type of a higher degree of individualization and a lower degree of developmental competence is produced. There are no exceptions to this generalization - not even the cancer cell. While a differentiated cell may become plastically deformed or necrobiotic, it can never form a new cell type through any means except the forward-moving course of cellular differentiation. Cellular reversion is a thermodynamic impossibility; it has never occurred and can never occur. Water will not run uphill - not even in cancer. The cancer cell is neither a deformed one nor a necrobiotic one. Its lethality resides in the very fact that intrinsically it is a normal cell - though its spatial and temporal relationship to the organism-as-a-whole is an abnormal one. The trophoblastic or unitarian thesis simply recognizes that:

1. the cancer cell is contained within the life-cycle and
2. that it is the most primitive cell in that life-cycle.

Though the diploid totipotent [stem] cells, which give origin to trophoblast, are known to be very abundant in the gonads, the question next arises as to their occurrence extra-genitally. Most modern pathologists[84] [85] [86] [87] [88] recognize the existence of so-called

---

[84] Boyd, W.: *Textbook of Pathology*, Lea & Febiger, ed. 4th, Philadelphia, 1943, p.309

[85] Ewing, J.: *Neoplastic Diseases*, Saunders, Philadelphia, 1940, p. 1045

ectopic germ cells (diploid totipotent cells) and Bounoure has, in an extensive monograph, recently reviewed the conclusive observational and experimental evidence for the dispersion of such cells throughout the soma.[89] Of course, embryologically, these cells are nothing more than totally undifferentiated cells that have not, as Arey phrased it, participated in body-building but have reserved their total potency or competency since the initial cleavage of the zygote.[90] Cells of various degrees of undifferentiation exist within the soma as a reservoir from which tissue repair and regeneration occur. *But only the totally undifferentiated cells of the soma are competent for meiosis;* these cells are the diploid totipotent [stem] cells. Of course, all cells in the soma are diploid, but only those that are *totally undifferentiated* are totally potent or *totipotent* - hence competent for meiosis. That such cells exist as well as function in the soma is further proven by the occasional occurrence of primary extra-genital chorionepithelioma in the male in such regions of low tissue reactivity as the pineal gland[91] [92] and the anterior mediastinum."[93] [94] [95] [96] The frankly exhibited trophoblast cells are correctly attributed to the only progenitor of trophoblast: a diploid totipotent cell that has undergone reduction division or meiosis to form a haploid gametogenous cell that has trophoblast formation as the only alternative to death [survival response].

Carcinogenesis is thus seen to be a phenomenon involving a spatially anomalous *differentiation* in response to organizer stimuli. (Primary uterine chorionepithelioma - as well as normal

---

[86] MacCallum, W.G.: *A. Textbook of Pathology*, ed. 4th, Saunders, Philadelphia, 1928, pp. 1087-1092

[87] Geist, S.H.: *Ovarian Tumors*, Paul B. Hoeber, New York, 1942, p.527

[88] Everett, N.B.: *J. Exp. Zool.* 92:49, 1943

[89] Bounoure, L.: *L'Origine des Cellules Reproductrices et le Problème de la Lignée Germinale*, Gauthier-Villars, Paris, 1939; *Continuité Germinale et Reproduction Agame*, ibid., 1940

[90] Arey, L.B.: *Developmental Anatomy*, ed. 3rd, Saunders, Philadelphia, 1934, p.10; cf. pp.71-76 ed. 4th.

[91] Glass, R.L. and Culbertson, S.A.: *Arch. Path.* 41:552, 1946

[92] Stowell, R.E., Sachs, E. and Russell, W.J.: *Am. J. Path.* 21:787, 1946

[93] Hirsch, O., Robbins, S.L. and Houghton, J.D.: *Am. J. Path.* 22:833, 1946

[94] Laipply, T.C. and Shipley, R.A.: *Am. J. Path.* 21:921, 1945

[95] Kantrowitz, A.R.: *Am. J. Path.* 10:531, 1934

[96] Schlumberger, H.G.: *Arch. Path.* 41:398, 1946

pregnancy trophoblast - while involving precisely the same differentiation in its origin, does not, of course, involve it anomalously.) The differentiation involves the phenomenon of meiosis with the consequent production of trophoblast, which, presented ectopically, is inevitably exhibited as cancer - the malignancy of which depends upon the extent to which such ectopic trophoblast is resisted. Thus in the unitarian thesis we see the malignant component in all exhibitions of cancer deriving from precisely the same cell type from which the chorionepitheliomas arise. We see all producing the same cell-type trophoblast. We see this cell doing ectopically precisely what it does in its normal canalization: eroding, infiltrating, and metastasizing.

"One of the most important problems in cancer research," Greenstein[97] points out, *"is concerned with the question of why primary tumors metastasize."* If cancer is trophoblastic, the problem of metastases is resolved: the normal pregnancy trophoblast is the *only* cell in the life-cycle that regularly metastasizes, doing so throughout the maternal host in the early months of pregnancy.[98] [99]

The stimuli to malignant differentiation are exemplified in the sex steroids, which induce the meiosis of diploid totipotent cells in their normal canalization. In view of the relatively specific organizer action of steroids, it is significant that practically all of the carcinogens are either steroids or, like diethylstilbestrol, possess the physiological properties of steroids. Though carcinogenesis may be mediated by highly diverse means, the ultimate common pathway involves the apposition of competent cell and organizer stimuli. The competent cell is always a totally undifferentiated cell (diploid totipotent [stem] cell) and the organizer stimulus ultimately involved appears to be a steroidal compound.

---

[97] Greenstein, J.P.: *Biochemistry of Cancer*, Academic Press, New York, 1947

[98] Schmorl, G.: *Verhandl. d. deutsch. path. Geselisch.* 2:39, 1904-1905; *Zentralbl. F. Gynak.* 29:129, 1905; cited by Yeit, later by Ewing, p. 638, and Park and Lees

[99] Veit, J.: *Ztschr. 1. Gebutish. u. Gynak.* 44:466, 1901

Agents producing a chronic inflammation can also prove indirectly carcinogenic, since chronic inflammatory sites have a marked capacity for localizing or concentrating steroidal sex hormones as well as other substances.[100] Certain chemicals may also prove indirectly carcinogenic through impairing the somatic detoxification mechanism for steroids.[101] [102] That under special and very limited circumstances viruses may also contribute to the common pathway by which malignant differentiation is accomplished in birds and rodents is recognized.[103] Virchow however pointed out 90 years ago that no stimulus can elicit from a tissue potencies not inherent within the tissue. The general consensus is that the role of the cancer virus is evocatory, eliciting from the organism an inherent potency; rather than creative, conferring *de novo* the cancer cell upon the organism.

ESTROGENS

Since the meiosis of normally canalized diploid totipotent cells is accomplished in both sexes through the organizer action of steroidal sex hormones, a review of the formidable literature on the carcinogenic properties of estrogen correlated with the unitarian thesis would be most pertinent to a complete elucidation of the thesis. Space will not permit this, and it must suffice to say that the normal estrogens bear as crucially a basic relationship to the origin of malignant cells, under ordinary circumstances, as chorionepithelioma bears to their cellular identity.

VIRUSES AND SOMATIC MUTATION

Since the virus theory is subsumed under the unitarian thesis - as a specialized contributory means[104] of eliciting the malignant

---

[100] Menkin, V.: *Dynamics of Inflammation*, Macmillan, New York, 1940

[101] Rusch, H. P., Baumann, C. A., Miller, J. A. and Kline, B. E.: in Symposium on Cancer, A.A.A.S. Research Conference on Cancer, ed. F. R. Moulton, Am. Assoc. Advancement of Science, Washington, W.C., 1945, p. 267.

[102] Gilbert, C. and Gillman, J.: *Science*. 99:398, 1944

[103] The phylogenic homologue of the trophoblast (extra-embryonic blastoderm) in birds is known to exhibit, under certain conditions, malignant properties: e.g., anidian formation (Edwards, C. L.: *Am. J. Physiol.* 6:351, 1902; cf. Ancel, P. and Vitemberger, P.: *Compt. rend. Soc. de Biol.* 92:172 and 1401, 1925; Grodzinski, Z.: *Archiv. f. Entwicklungsmechanik.* 129:502, 1933; 131:653, 1934)

[104] Joseph Needham has cogently remarked: "It is an instructive exercise to read through the writings on the virus theory of cancer substituting the words 'active

differentiation - the chief remaining theory is the somatic mutation hypothesis. This hypothesis explains nothing and is, in fact, little more than a circular definition: cancer is due to a change; a change is a mutation. This change occurs in the body or soma; therefore, cancer is due to a somatic mutation. On the other hand, the trophoblastic or unitarian thesis does embrace a very definite genetic "mutation." This "mutation" is expressed as meiosis whereby, with the division of the consequent gametogenous cell, the ectopic trophoblast (cancer) cell presented to the soma is, through the necessity of meiosis, *of a genetic composition unique from the soma;* and, therefore, in the most literal, genetic sense, a neoplasm.

Even were one uncritically to accept the somatic mutation hypothesis[105] or the virus theory of cancer,[106] it would be necessary either to seek their resolution in the unitarian or trophoblastic thesis or to turn to a non-unitarian explanation. In which case it would be necessary then to postulate an indefinitely large variety of unknown cancer viruses or a similar variety of unknown somatic mutations to account for the origin of the cancer cell. But not even these would suffice since neither hypothesis could account for the fiercely malignant behavior of normal trophoblast *in vitro* - nor for the fact that this cell has never been found in a non-pregnant organism except as cancer.

MEIOSIS

We have observed that the extra-genital dispersion of diploid totipotent cells is a commonplace fact. We have specifically ascribed the origin of all morphological exhibitions of cancer to the meiosis of one or more such diploid totipotent cells with the consequent production of a gametogenous cell, whose only alternative to death is division with the resulting production of trophoblast.

---

agent' or 'active extract' for 'virus' wherever it occurs. The results are illuminating." (Needham, J.: *Biochemistry and Morphogenesis*, Cambridge Univ. Press, 1942, p. 268)

[105] Haldane, J. B. S.: *J. Path. and Bact.* 38:507, 1934

[106] Maisin, J.: *Cancer II Radiations-Virus Environment*, Casterman, Tournai - Paris, 1949; cf. Duran-Reynals, F., *Am. J. Med.* 8.490-511, 1950.

In the normal reproductive canalization the *only* way in which trophoblast can arise is through the meiosis of a diploid totipotent cell and the consequent division (non-sexually or by fertilization) of the resulting gametogenous cell to produce trophoblast. Therefore, one question alone remains here: can the same diploid totipotent cell in an extragenital site undergo meiosis to eventuate in trophoblast production?

As early as 1879 Arnold observed gametoid (meiotic) mitosis in malignant tissue. About twenty years later Farmer, Moore and Walker reported the occurrence of meiosis (heterotypic mitosis) at the border of malignant tumors.[107] In 1929 Evans and Swezy described in inflamed somatic tissue changes "strikingly similar to those of meiotic mitosis."[108] In 1936 Hearne observed meiotic changes in tissues cultured with methylcholanthrene,[109] and Molenorff made similar observations in 1939 with estrone.[110]

Diploid totipotent cells are dispersed throughout the soma. Meiosis occurs within the soma. Frank trophoblast cells occur within the soma - though inevitably in a malignant exhibition. They can arise only through the division of a gametogenous cell produced by the meiosis of a diploid totipotent cell. Frank trophoblast cells have never been found in the soma except as the most malignant exhibition of cancer - with the exception of pregnancy.

Indeed, the difficulty is no longer one of accounting for the origin of the definitive malignant cell through the phenomena discussed, but rather one of seeking *any* explanation of how the meiosis of ectopic diploid totipotent cells, exposed to adequate organizer stimuli, could invariably be averted so as to preclude their normal differentiation to trophoblast, whose ectopic exhibition has never been known except in a malignant fashion. Frankly exhibited, such trophoblast comprises the most malignant exhibition of cancer possible, though when morphologically masked by the somatic

---

[107] Farmer, J. B., Moore, J. E., Walker, C. E.: *Lancet* 2:1830, 1903; *B.M.J.* 2:1664, 1903
[108] Evans H. M. and Swezy, O.: *Memoirs.of Univ. Calif.* 9:1-65, 1929
[109] Hearne, E. M., *Nature*, 138:291, 1936
[110] Molendorff, W. v.: *Klin. Wchnschr.* 18:1089, 1939

response of the hostal cells, the malignancy of such trophoblast is moderated.

UNITARIAN VS. NON UNITARIAN THESIS

The body of experimentally established facts comprising modern oncology is formidable. It is not possible for any explicitly defined thesis to stand unless it is congruent with, or at least not contradictory to, such facts. Only the unitarian thesis finds such congruence. To the unitarian thesis in general and in particular to the preceding data outlined for it, it is especially instructive to apply Herbert Spencer's criterion of truth - the inconceivability of the opposite. The thesis opposite or alternative to the unitarian one is that each morphological exhibition of cancer represents a biologically distinctive phenomenon, each with a malignant component different from all others. <u>This would mean literally hundreds of basically different types of cancer cells</u> - each type being normally unrepresented in the life cycle; therefore, each being spontaneously created. Not only would it become necessary to postulate the existence of hundreds of distinct species of cancer cells, but also a postulate of an almost infinite number of subspecies of each type of cancer cell would be required to account for the varying degrees of malignancy exhibited by a given malignant lesion in the course of its evolution. Since a single chemical carcinogen can evoke practically any malignant exhibition, then it would become necessary, according to any non-unitarian concept, to conclude that causes which are alike produce effects that are unlike. On the same basis, the occurrence of the frankly exhibited trophoblast cells of extra-genital chorionepithelioma in the male (identical with those of the primary uterine form) would necessitate the unbiological conclusion that cells which are alike arise from cells that are unlike. The logical negation of *any* non-unitarian hypothesis is further apparent in the experimentally defined uniformity of cancer cells in every one of over twenty factors studied to date. (pp.1-2 of this thesis)

In contrast to the alternative non-unitarian hypothesis, the unitarian thesis holds that the malignant component in all exhibitions of cancer is the same; that this component is not spontaneously created but represents the most primitive cell in the life-cycle; that this cell arises not through "reversion" but through

98

differentiation; that the varying morphological exhibitions are simply conditioned by the nature and resistance of the tissue in which the ectopic trophoblast finds itself; and that the malignancy of the exhibition is, roughly, expressed in the degree of deformation of the somatic tissue by the ectopic trophoblast - and that this is reflected in the morphology from which histological diagnoses derive.

The unitarian thesis and the trophoblastic thesis are of logical necessity synonymous: the most malignant exhibition of cancer (chorionepithelioma) comprises cells intrinsically identical with pregnancy trophoblast cells.[111] Then, if cancer is a unitarian phenomenon, the malignant component of the varying morphological types must be trophoblastic; for, two quantities equal to a third are equal to each other.

Finally, were we to set aside all else evidential of the unitarian or trophoblastic nature of cancer, and scrutinize but a single datum, we should find that neither experimental fact nor scientific reasoning can offer any alternative to the trophoblastic nature of cancer in explanation. This one datum is the fact that many authors over the past half-century have described frank trophoblast (chorionepithelioma) metastasizing from a primary site to appear at the secondary site in an adenocarcinomatous or other exhibition.[112] [113] [114] And the converse has frequently been seen.[115] Moreover, frankly exhibited trophoblast (chorionepithelioma) often has been described as merging by imperceptible degrees into an adenocarcinomatous or sarcomatous exhibition. In their

---

[111] The malignant exhibition of the trophoblast of the placenta is the expression of a lack of extrinsic growth restraints against the trophoblast [enzyme activity]; this fact was demonstrated in the tissue culture of normal rabbit trophoblast.

[112] Ewing, J.: *Neoplastic Diseases*, Saunders, Philadelphia, 1940, p. 90, p. 863

[113] Ahlstrom, C. C.: *Acta path. et microbiol. Scandinav.* 8:231, 1931

[114] Molotoff, W. G.: Virchow's *Arch. f. path.* 288.317-325, 1933; cf. Da Silva Horta, J. and Madeira, F.: *Arch. espan. urol.* 2:350, 1946; cf. Gaertner, K., *Frankfurt. Ztsch. f. Path.* 52:1, 1938; Willis, Rupert A.: *The Spread of Tumors in the Human Body*, J. A. Churchill, London, 1934, p. 134 [cf. p. 164, "Cancer, a Composite Tissue"]

[115] Brewer, J. I.: *Arch. Path.* 41:580, 1946; Cf. (4l): Cf.   Stewart, M. J.: *J. Path.* 17:409, 1912

comprehensive monograph on chorionepithelioma, Park and Lees (1950) write:

"There is no doubt that in many instances of testicular chorionepithelioma, certainly in several of our sections, characteristic trophoblast merges imperceptibly with areas of undifferentiated tissue whose hostal origin would never be questioned." [116]

THE TROPHOBLAST AND THE PANCREAS

John Beard, a lecturer in embryology at the University of Edinburgh, first published on the trophoblastic thesis of cancer in June, 1902.[117] By February 1905, he reported, on embryological grounds, the antithesis of the pancreatic enzymes to the trophoblast cell;[118] and, a few years later he specifically pointed out that the cancer or trophoblast cell protected itself against pancreatic enzymes through the production of specific antitryptic substances.[119] The occurrence of tryptic inhibitors in cancer sera has, during the past forty years, been described by at least fifteen different workers,[120] though not within the context of the trophoblastic thesis.

---

[116] Park, W. W. and Lees, J. C.: *Arch. Path.* 49:73-104, 205-241, 1950

[117] Beard, J.: *Lancet* 1: 1758, 1902

[118] Beard, J.: *Lancet* 1:281, 1905

[119] Beard, J.: "The Enzyme Treatment of Cancer and Its Scientific Basis - Being Collected Papers Dealing with the Origin, Nature and Scientific Treatment of the Natural Phenomenon Known as Malignant Disease", Chatto & Windus, London, 1911, p. 204

[120] Brieger, L. and Trebing, J.: *Berlin klin. Wchnschr.*, 45:1041; 1349; 2260, 1908; Bergmann, V. and Bamberg, K.: *Berlin klin. Wchnschr.* 45: 1396, 1908; Schultz, W. and Chiarolanza,. R.: *Deutsche Med. Wchnsch.* 34:1300, 1908; Herzfeld, E.: *Berlin klin. Wchnschr.* 45..2182, 1908.1; Orszag, O. and Barcza, A.: *Orvosi hetilap.* No. 34, 1909; Brenner, F.: *Deutche med. Wchnschr.*, 35:390 1909; Torday, A.: *Budapesti orvosi, ujsag* No. 35, 1909; Schlorlemmer, R. and Selter,...: *Ztschr. f. klin. Med.* 69: 153, 1910; Veechi, A.: *Riforma med.* 26:1158; 1188, 1910; *abstr. Wien. klin. Wchnschr.* 24:- 216, 1911; Guthmann, H. and Hess, L.: *Arch. f. Gynak.* 131:462, 1928; Clark, D. G., Clifton,E. E. and Newton, B. L.: *Proc. Soc. Exper. Biol. and Med.* 69:276, 1948; West, P. M. and Hilliard, J.: *Ann. West. Med. and Surg.* 3:227, 1949; Cliffton, E. E.: *J. Natl. Cancer Institute*, 10:719, 1949; Dillard, G. H. and Chanutin, A.: *Cancer Research* 9:665, 1949; West, P. M.: *Cancer Research* 10:248, 1950; Waldvogel, M. Marvin, H. and Wells, B.: *Proc. Soc. Exper.. Biol. and Med.* 72-100, 1949

In 1947, Krebs, Krebs and Gurchot first pointed out the specific antithesis of chymotrypsin to the malignant (or trophoblast) cell.[121] In 1948 Clark, Cliffton and Newton further confirmed the specific antitryptic antithesis of the cancer cell and offered evidence for the diagnostic and prognostic utilization of the phenomenon. In 1949, West and Hilliard, in the study of the sera of over 3,000 cancer patients, reported the specific antithesis of the malignant cell to chymotrypsin by showing that 15 grams of crystalline chymotrypsin would be necessary - in a single dose - to neutralize all of the *average excess of* chymotrypsin inhibitor in the serum of the advanced cancer patient. The latter workers proposed the utilization of the specific antichymotryptic titer of the serum for prognostic but not necessarily diagnostic purpose.[122] [123]

It is noteworthy that West and Hilliard, as well as others, have described a quantitative relationship between the concentration of cancer cells and the titer of specific chymotrypsin inhibitor. This titer was observed to fall after the surgical removal of the malignant tumor and to rise linearly with its recurrence. Thus the data on the antitryptic properties of cancer sera are not only proof of the antithesis between the cancer cell and the pancreatic enzymes, but are further evidential of the unitarian - and thereby atrophoblastic - nature of cancer.

Since the malignant cell is not spontaneously created but has its normal counterpart in the most primitive cell of the life-cycle, each organism in the span of its own gestation destroys the cellular counterpart of cancer. This destruction is accomplished through the pancreatic enzymes, notably chymotrypsin and amylase.

When the mammalian organism totally fails in this, the pregnancy trophoblast overgrows as chorionepithelioma.[124] A partial failure is

---

[121] Krebs, E. T., Krebs, E. T., Jr. and Gurchot, C.: *M. Rec.* 160: 479, 1947

[122] West, P. M. and Hilliard, J.: *Ann. West. Med. And Surg.* 3:227, 1949

[123] West, P. M.: *Cancer Research*, 10:248, 1950

[124] Mueller, C. W. and Lapp, W. A.: *Am. J. Obst. and Gynec.* 58:133, 1949; cf. *Obst and Gynec. Survey* 5:102, 1950 for excellent commentary

reflected as a toxemic pregnancy,[125] and/or a hydatidiform mole accompanied by an abnormally high excretion of chorionic (trophoblastic) gonadotrophin. For this reason hydatidiform moles are most frequently associated with toxemic pregnancies, while the risk of sequent chorionepithelioma is 2,000 to 4,000 times greater after hydatidiform mole than after normal pregnancy.[126]   The reason for *"the much higher curability rate of choriocarcinoma preceded by hydatidiform mole,"* as reported by Park and Lees, [127] is that the precedent hydatidiform mole represented at least a partially successful antithesis on the part of the maternal host to the trophoblast.

The reason why primary uterine chorionepithelioma can, within a few weeks, arise and kill the patient is that this most malignant tumor simply represents *a hyperplasia* of normal trophoblast cells freed from their extrinsic restraint - just as the *in vitro* culture of the rabbit trophoblast freed from the maternal environment yields a fiercely malignant exhibition.

It is well established:[128]

1. that pregnant diabetics exhibit a greatly increased incidence of the pregnancy toxemias;
2. that the severity of such toxemias varies directly with the overgrowth of cellular trophoblast as reflected in the abnormally elevated excretion of chorionic gonadotrophin;
3. that the phenomenon involves a non-insulin deficiency of the pancreas gland;
4. that the predisposition to pregnancy toxemias is noted as early as five years prior to the clinical onset of diabetes;[129] [130]

[125] Krebs, E. T., Jr. and Bartlett, C. L.: *M. Rec.* 162:1, 1949
[126] Park, W. W. and Lees, J. C.: *Arch. Path.* 49:73-104, 1950; cf. pp. 75, 81
[127] Park, W. W. and Lees, J. C.: *Arch. Path.* 49:73-104, 1950; cf. pp. 75, 81
[128] The complete bibliography for these data is given in Krebs & Bartlett's monograph on "The Pregnancy Toxemias, the Role of the Trophoblast and the Pancreas" *M. Rec.* 162, 1949
[129] Stromme, W. B.: *Journal-Lancet* 70:13, 1950
[130] Miller, H. C., Hurwitz, D. and Kinder, K.: *J. A. M. A.* 124: 271, 1941

5. that the administration of steroidal sex hormones in such pregnancy toxemias frequently ameliorates the condition; and

6. that this amelioration is reflected in a proportionate depression in the urinary excretion of chorionic gonadotrophin.

Since such steroidal sex hormones as estrogen depress the proliferation of cellular trophoblast both in normal and toxemic pregnancies, as reflected in a depression in the urinary excretion of chorionic (cytotrophoblastic) gonadotrophin, it is significant that Kullander (1948) found in the primary uterine chorionepithelioma that the administration of stilbestrol resulted in a clinical improvement that paralleled the decline in the urinary excretion of chorionic gonadotrophin.[131] Though Kullander did not cure his patients, so long as stilbestrol controlled the excretion of chorionic gonadotrophin, they improved.

It is a commonplace observation that the administration of estrogen or testosterone during pregnancy will often depress the production of chorionic gonadotrophin sufficiently to cause the Aschheim-Zondek test or its Friedman modification to become negative.

In listing the criteria of malignancy, Oberling and Woglom write: *"...above all is the impudent independence called autonomy."*[132] Certainly, no other property is more characteristic of the cancer cell than autonomy; *yet in the most malignant exhibition of cancer possible we find the trophoblast cells showing the same susceptibility to the checking influence of sex steroids as is found for the normal pregnancy trophoblast.*

If cancer is trophoblastic, and as such a unitarian phenomenon, it would seem that the steroidal sex hormones should suppress the growth not only of pregnancy trophoblast and chorionepithelioma but all other exhibitions of cancer as well. That this would be the

---

[131] Kullander, S.: *Lancet* 1:944, 1948

[132] Oberling, C. (trans. by Wm. H. Woglom): *The Riddle of Cancer*, Yale Univ. Press, New Haven, 1944

case were sufficient localization of the steroidal sex hormones possible at all malignant sites is shown in the fact that these hormones do act to suppress the growth of mammary cancer, prostatic cancer, and their metastases involving the skeletal system. Morphologically, the difference between a primary mammary cancer and a prostatic one is much less pronounced than the difference between either and a primary chorionepithelioma.

The placenta, the prostate, and the mammary gland are notably capable of the selective localization of steroids; hence, trophoblast in any of these areas will show a like response to the injection of steroidal sex hormones. In the case of prostatic and mammary growths the use of the physiologically antagonistic steroid is rational, since such causes the somatic elements in the growth to atrophy. That the palliative effect is dependent upon the ability of the *somatic* elements in the tumor to localize the steroids is shown in the fact that the skeletal metastases from the prostate as well as from the mammary gland are responsive specifically to estrogen and testosterone, respectively. Yet this amenability is lost as, with increasing malignancy, the original somatic elements in the skeletal metastases are lost. That such a loss is not directly due to the increasing malignancy but indirectly to the loss of the specific somatic cells responsible for the localization of the steroids is indicated by the fact that in the placenta, while the localizing somatic elements remain, the growth of the vastly more malignant chorionepitheliomatous exhibition is checked.

Thus we find the unitarian principle of cancer implicit in the sex hormone therapy of cancer, as in all other useful forms of cancer therapy. Moreover, in the unitarian principle the use of steroidal sex hormones in cancer finds its first rationale.

Since a non-insulin pancreatic deficiency has been identified with the overgrowth of pregnancy trophoblast, which overgrowth has been shown amenable to steroidal sex hormones, two questions arise:

1. what is the nature of the deficient pancreatic factor, and
2. is the deficiency of this factor associated with the overgrowth of *all* trophoblast?

About half a century ago John Beard found a concomitance between the commencing function of the fetal pancreas, as indicated by the appearance of zymogen granules in the gland, and the precipitate degeneration of the trophoblast or its phylogenetic homologue.[133] Broad comparative studies confirmed his thesis that, in the span of normal gestation, the pancreatic enzymes are responsible for checking the growth and ultimately destroying the gestational trophoblast or its homologue. In fact, Beard's studies were so carefully performed that he was able to state half a century ago that in the 56th day in the span of human gestation, the cellular trophoblast undergoes a sudden degeneration. Some 30 years after this work, the trophoblast cell-produced chorionic gonadotrophin was discovered, and only recently has the quantitative technique for the estimation of chorionic gonadotrophin been sufficiently perfected to show that a composite[134] excretion curve for chorionic gonadotrophin made through the span of human gestation coincides precisely with the curve predicted half a century ago by John Beard.[135]

If the urinary excretion of chorionic gonadotrophin persists at the original level after the 56th to 70th day in the span of human gestation, the process is inevitably exhibited as chorionepithelioma. In fact, if the abnormal elevation of chorionic gonadotrophin found in pancreatic dysfunction in pregnancy exceeds a certain level, again the process is exhibited as chorionepithelioma.

In view of the antithesis of the pancreatic proteases to the trophoblast cell, it is clear why both pregnancy and cancer are associated with high titers of trypsin and chymotrypsin inhibitors: antithesis is a two-way street, so to speak.

---

[133] Beard, J.: Anat. Anz. 8:22, 1892; *Nature* 47:79, 1892; Beard, J.: On Certain Problems of Vertebrate Embryology, G. Fischer, Jena, 1896, 78 pp; Beard, J.: The Span of Gestation and the Cause of Birth, G. Fischer, Jena, 1897, 132 pp.; Beard, J.: *Anat Anz.* 18:465, 1900; Beard, J.: *Anat Anz.* 21:50, 1902; Beard, J.: *Anat Anz.* 21:189, 1902; Beard, J.: *Berlin klin Wchnschr.* 40:- 695, 1903; Beard, J.: *Lancet* 2:1200, 1904

[134] Beard, J.: *Anat. Anz.* 8:22, 1892; *Nature* 47:79, 1892

[135] Patten, B. M.: *Human Embryology*, Blakiston & Company, Philadelphia, 1946, p. 173

If the pancreatic enzymes are antithetic to the cancer cell, if they resist the cancer cell as the cancer cell is known to resist them (through the specific antitryptic inhibitors) why does cancer of the pancreas gland occur? Why is it that cancer is not only primary in this gland but that this gland itself may be subject to secondary growths through metastases or direct invasion?

The pancreatic proteases exist in the pancreas in the form of their *inactive* zymogens. These are not converted into the corresponding active enzymes until they are acted upon by the kinases of the blood or, especially, by those of the small intestine. In view of this, one may ask why the small intestine, then, is not practically immune to cancer. Woglom answers this question well in his commentary in an abstract of a paper by Raab:

"One of the most striking features about the pathology of malignant disease is the almost complete absence of carcinoma in the duodenum and its increasing frequency throughout the gastrointestinal tract in direct proportion to the distance from this exempt segment." [136]

It is noteworthy that the small intestine is not only practically immune to primary tumors, but also to metastases. A fulminating malignant growth may exist in the pyloric end of the stomach a few millimeters from the immune small intestine, but, as William Boyd points out, *"The duodenum is never invaded, the tumor stopping short at the pylorus. Spread to neighboring organs usually involves the liver or the pancreas."* [137] The incidence of malignancy is, of course, high immediately distal to the ileocecal valve.

The pancreatic enzymes not only normally occur in the active state in the blood stream which possesses an optimum pH for their action but the clinical determination of serum amylase and trypsin are standard procedures, especially in pancreatic diseases.

---

[136] Raab, W.: *Klin Wchnschr.* 14:1633, 1935
[137] Boyd, W.: *Textbook of Pathology*, Lea & Febiger, Philadelphia, 1943, p. 488

THE PANCREAS AND CARCINOGENESIS

The fact that pregnancy occurs in the presence of a normal concentration of pancreatic enzymes indicates that trophoblast can exist for a while under such conditions. It must be remembered, however, that such trophoblast is: (1) held in check until the 56th day of gestation and almost completely destroyed shortly thereafter (with the commencing function of the fetal pancreas) and (2) that implantation occurs *after* the trophoblast has had about a four-day period of growth anatomically exterior to the host.

The trophoblast carries with it its own antitryptic enzymes against the pancreatic proteases. As we have seen, *carcinogenesis involves ectopically precisely the same basic mechanisms involved in the production of canalized trophoblast.* The prolonged exposure of a tissue to carcinogens results in a prolonged depression in its respiratory mechanisms.[138] This may result in the appearance and persistence of ectopic trophoblast in the exposed tissue. The trophoblast or cancer cell is autonomous of the hostal respiratory system and is obligatively anaerobic, undergoing aerobic glycolysis even in the presence of a free oxygen.[139] The trophoblastic thesis explains the long-known identity of trophoblast cell metabolism with that of the cancer cell: an obligative anaerobic system is obviously a necessity in a primitive parasitic cell like the trophoblast (or cancer) cell.[140] [141] [142]

When cancer is elicited experimentally from a normal laboratory animal, the lesion usually does not metastasize, but attains a large size and is almost completely somatic. Herein reside the scientific limitations of artificially induced or transplanted animal tumors in the scientific study of chemotherapeutic agents. Such tumors are practically benign in a biological sense. Because the pregnancy trophoblast regularly and normal metastasizes in the early phase of

---

[138] Boyland, E.: *Biochem. J.* 27:791, 1933

[139] Needham, J.: *Chemical Embryology,* Cambridge, 1931, Op. 1461, 771

[140] Bell, W. B., Cunningham, L., Jowett, M., Millet, H. and Brooks, J.: *Brit. M. J.* 1:126, 1928

[141] Cramer, William: *The Metabolism of the Trophoblast in Studies on the Diagnosis and Nature of Cancer,* William Wood & Company, New York, p. 125

[142] Loeser, A.: *Arch. f. Gynak.* 148:118, 1932; *Centralbl. f. Gynak.* 56:206, 1932

gestation, we must expect metastases ultimately in any "full blown" cancer.

While a low-grade malignant growth (primarily somatic tumefaction) can be induced ultimately by sufficient carcinogenic stimuli in the presence of normal pancreatic function, a highly malignant exhibition is invariably accompanied by at least a relative pancreatic insufficiency implicit in the correspondingly high serum titer of antitryptic and antichymotryptic enzymes.

That the induction of the ectopic trophoblast is usually accomplished against great difficulty - regardless of pancreatic adequacy - is indicated in the fact that non-chorionepitheliomatous exhibitions in man usually have a latent period of years, while a chorionepithelioma in pregnancy may arise from the pre-existing trophoblast and destroy the host within a few weeks.

The extent to which the soma resists malignant involution is reflected in the fact that only two cellular differentiations - meiosis of the diploid totipotent cell and subsequent division of the resultant gametogenous cell - divide the malignant cell from the benign one. This explains the all-or-none suddenness classic to the malignant change - and the absence of true transitional cells.

CANCER A COMPOSITE TISSUE
The malignant lesion is a composite tissue comprising (1) trophoblast plus (2) somatic elements. The malignancy of a lesion varies directly with its concentration of trophoblast and inversely with its concentration of somatic elements. The normal placenta, too, represents a composite tissue; for here the trophoblast cell finds its normal canalization in the life-cycle. Just as the malignancy of a placenta, in a chorionepitheliomatous exhibition, varies directly with the concentration of trophoblast cells, so in the ectopic presentation of trophoblast that comprises cancer the malignancy of the lesion varies with its concentration of trophoblast. The only fundamental difference is that in the latter the trophoblast cells are morphologically masked by the resisting soma - except in the most malignant of genital tumors: chorionepithelioma.

108

A tissue can be malignant only by being a composite one. Malignancy is an antithetic relationship between cells and finds being by virtue of a thetic benignancy. In its simplest terms then, a malignant tumor comprises somatic tumefaction plus a malignant component. It is for this reason that the greatest tumefaction is usually associated with the least malignant exhibitions and the least tumefaction often with the most malignant exhibitions.

Since trophoblast normally metastasizes, tumors of the highest malignancy and lowest tumefaction tend to be the most metastatic. Thus the increase or decrease in the malignancy of a given tumor is not the result of a continuing spontaneous generation of an infinite variety of cancer cells, *but merely the expression of the increase or decrease in the concentration of* A CONSTANT MALIGNANT COMPONENT. As the antithesis of this component determines the malignancy of the lesion so the soma determines its benignancy.

LEUKEMIA
In the leukemias the constant malignant component (trophoblast) is present in the lymphopoietic or myelopoietic tissues. The reaction of such tissues to the malignant component results in the proliferation of *somatic* white blood cells of varying degrees of maturity. This is the counterpart of tumefaction in the sessile tumor. Thus the unitarian or trophoblastic thesis, different from the non-unitarian concept, finds no contradiction in the fact that often the most malignant phase of the leukemic process - the so-called aleukemic leukemia - actually involves a leukopenia. This phase is the most malignant because the somatic cells (leukopoietic tissue) have lost their ability to resist through virtue of the destruction of the leukopoietic tissue by ectopic trophoblast. For this reason the aleukemic or leukopenic stage is often terminal to a preceding highly leukemic or leukocytic phase.

TROPHOBLASTIC HORMONES
The routine utilization of the trophoblastic hormone, chorionic gonadotrophin, is of course a clinical commonplace as a means of diagnosis as an index to therapeutic response in the case of the most malignant exhibitions of cancer - the chorionepitheliomas and certain other exhibitions of cancer. The excretion of this hormone

varies directly with the malignancy of the tumor, which, in turn, varies directly with the concentration of trophoblast cells.

In 1944 Roffo[143] reported a similar gonadotrophin in all of 1,000 cancer patients examined, and none in the blood or urine of the control series, with the exception of pregnancy, of course. In 1946 Krebs and Gurchot reported the identification of Roffo's gonadotrophin as trophoblastic.[144] In 1947 Beard, Halperin and Liebert published a confirmation of the prior papers and suggested a practical utilization of the phenomenon.[145] Prior to these studies, numerous scattered reports of chorionic gonadotrophin in cancer serum and urine appeared in the literature, yet without the context of any unified theory. Zondek reported the hormone in the urine of 82 per cent of females afflicted with cancers of the genital organs and in 36 per cent of female patients suffering from extra-genital tumors.[146] [147] Five years later, Zondek was able to duplicate and extend his original findings,[148] which had been confirmed by others.[149]

It is necessary to emphasize that the original work of Zondek as well as other workers was done on the erroneous assumption that the hormone was produced by the anterior pituitary gland. Even after tissue culture studies had proved the trophoblast-cell-origin of the hormone, its occasional identification in cancer urines, through the use of the Ascheim-Zondek or Friedman tests, was usually dismissed as an inexplicable datum of an inexplicable disease. Only within the context of the unitarian or trophoblastic thesis was sufficient theoretical justification found to concentrate and selectively extract the urines of the less malignant exhibitions of

[143] Roffo, A.: *Bol. inst. de med. exper. para el estud. v. trat. d. cancer.* 21:419, 1944
[144] Krebs, E. T., Jr. and Gurchot, C.: *Science* 104:302, 1946
[145] Beard, H., Halperin, B. and Liebert, S.: *Science* 105:475, 1947
[146] Zondek, B.: *Klin Wchtschr.*, 9:679, 1930
[147] Zondek, B.: *Chirurg.* 2:1072, 1930
[148] Zondek, B.: *Hormone des Ovariums und des Hypophysenvorderlappens,* Springe, Vienna, 1935
[149] Laquer, F., Dottl, K. and Friedrich, H.: *Medizin und Chemie* 2:117, 1934; cf. Laquer, W. A.: *J. Obst. Gynaec. Brit. Emp.* 52:468, 1945; De Fermo, C.: *Arch. ital. chir.* 33:801, 1933; *abstr. Ztschr. f. Krebsforsch.* 40: Ref. 96,1934; Valasquez, J. and Engel, P.: *Endocrinology* 27:523, 1940

cancer specifically for the same hormones (chorionic gonadotrophin and syncytial steroids), always found by ordinary techniques in the most malignant exhibitions.

Thus to the already established uniformities for 20 or more known factors among the various exhibitions of cancer, we now find a hormone (not only evidential of the unitarian thesis but of the specific trophoblastic nature of cancer as well) in the trophoblast cell-produced hormones. *Like all other uniformities found in the malignant lesion* that for the trophoblastic hormones becomes increasingly apparent with the malignancy of the growth, so that frank chorionepitheliomas are found excreting as many as one million International Units of chorionic gonadotrophin every 24 hours, while the much less malignant exhibitions with no frank trophoblast cells excrete 50 or fewer units of the trophoblastic hormone.

DIAGNOSTIC IMPLICATIONS
There are only two fundamental kinds of cancer tests:

1. the indirect tests concerned with the detection of a substance produced *by the soma* as the result of the presence of cancer cells; and
2. the direct tests concerned with the detection of a substance produced by the cancer cells themselves.

Though the incidence of a specific somatic change may bear a high correlation with the presence of a uniform stimulus, the correlation can never be a truly specific one, since obviously no *somatic* reaction is so specifically reserved for the presence of cancer or trophoblast cells that it can not be falsely elicited by other stimuli.

The limitations of the indirect tests have been demonstrated in practice. The only reliable and generally accepted serum or urine tests for cancer are the direct ones, such as the Ascheim-Zondek test and its numerous modifications. Just as hundreds of indirect tests have been tried and discarded for pregnancy diagnosis, so have hundreds of indirect tests for cancer been tried and then discarded. The only tests for either pregnancy or cancer that have survived are those *direct* tests depending upon the identification of a substance unique to cancer and pregnancy: the hormone of the trophoblast cell. Since cancer is trophoblastic, its most malignant exhibition – chorionepithelioma - is highly amenable to the direct test. In fact, the possibility of either an indirect or direct general diagnostic test for cancer depends upon cancer being a unitarian phenomenon.

The efficient clinical implementation of the trophoblastic or unitarian thesis depends upon the development of a simple, reliable and highly accurate quantitative test for the specific products of the trophoblast cell. While we have identified the presence of chorionic gonadotrophin in the urines of patients with all exhibitions of cancer, we have found the technological evolution of a quantitatively precise chorionic gonadotrophin test difficult for the less malignant exhibitions of cancer. When we consider that a chorionepitheliomatous exhibition of cancer in the male may yield over 1,000,000 IU of chorionic gonadotrophin while metastatic testicular cancers of a much lower malignancy - though biologically still more malignant than most extragenital growths - may yield fewer than 50 IU for a like volume of urine, then the physical difficulties in the case of most of the extragenital tumors of still lower malignancy are obvious.

From the urines of patients with the common exhibitions of cancer, the authors have obtained highly active preparations of chorionic gonadotrophin, and are now engaged in the crystallization of chorionic gonadotrophin, by the method of Claesson, Hogberg and Westman, from pooled urines of various exhibitions of cancer.[150] It is recognized that the specific steroidal hormones of the syncytial trophoblast also comprise a most important avenue to the development of a satisfactory diagnostic technique. However, these steroidal hormones have not been studied as intensely as chorionic gonadotrophin, which is now characterized as a gluco-protein containing 18 per cent acetylglucosaminedigalactose polysaccharide.

---

[150] Claesson, L., Hogberg, B., Rosenberg, Th. and Westman, A.: *Acta Endocrnol.* 1:1-48,1948

Several cancer tests relying on the detection of trophoblastic hormones are now under study for the purpose of achieving a sufficiently practical quantitative test for general use.

CLINICAL IMPLICATION

As a composite tissue, cancer in its somatic component represents many diseases; in its constant malignant component, one disease; and, in its totality, a local manifestation of a general disease. Since the perspective of the clinician is necessarily anthropomorphic, he sees cancer primarily in its somatic phase as a series of many diseases. On the other hand, as Oberling and Woglom have so aptly phrased it, *"To the experimentalist cancer is one disease and one disease only."*

Both clinician and experimentalist are generally agreed that the somatic or anatomical changes produced by the malignant process are largely irreversible. Surgical extirpation or the primarily non-selective cautery of radiant energy may destroy the composite tissue of a primary tumor. But the vague hope for an agent that will cause the "reversion" of an organized malignant tumor to normal tissue is scientifically indefensible. Aside from the physical destruction of the tumor itself, one primary factor can contribute to the amelioration of the effect of the tumor on the host. This is the growth inhibition or destruction of the constant malignant component of the tumor. Selective ablation of the malignant component will not alter the already existing somatic dysplasia nor histologically change the architectonics of the tumor, except in highly malignant anaplastic exhibitions. Here the histological as well as the gross changes take an expected course: an histological increase in connective tissue elements with a palpable increase in fibrosity.

In the advanced and well organized lesion, the possible changes are not, as a rule, dramatic. Were the malignant component ablated, the somatic component would tend to persist largely unchanged, or even show a slight increase in benign tumefaction. Since none of the cells in a malignant tumor is *per se* a "diseased" or pathological cell, but rather a cell normal to the life-cycle, cancer does not itself produce any "toxic effects."[151] Its lethality is eminently a physical matter involving the normal behavior of normal trophoblast in a spatially abnormal relationship.

Above all, cancer is a natural phenomenon ultimately involving the soma in irreversible changes. To question the results expected from the selective ablation of the constant malignant component in a malignant lesion would be to suggest that, aside from actual tumor destruction, no malignant tumor has ever spontaneously regressed, that no highly anaplastic cancer has even spontaneously gone into a less malignant scirrhous exhibition, or that no patient has ever survived for five years or more after exhibiting an inoperable and highly malignant lesion. It is not necessary to review here an impressive literature on spontaneous regression. Much more important to a sound comprehension of the clinical implications of the trophoblastic or unitarian thesis are the thousands of cases of cancer in which the host is able to resist and to live with the cancer cells for years.

- What are the factors - cells, tissues, organs, and their secretions – contributing to such resistance?
- What causes trophoblast in the pregnant diabetic to overgrow, despite a normal insulin supplement?
- Why do the specific inhibitors to pancreatic chymotrypsin and trypsin rise with the increasing malignancy of a growth and decline following its amelioration?
- Why is the small intestine practically immune not only to primary tumors, but to direct invasion and metastases as well?
- Why does the growth of the invasive, erosive and metastatic trophoblast of normal gestation cease and degeneration commence concomitant with the commencing function of the fetal pancreas gland?

---

[151] The answers to these questions reflect the cogency of Oberling's prediction: "Some day perhaps, it will turn out to be one of the ironies of nature that cancer, responsible for so many deaths, should be so indissolubly connected with life." (Oberling, C. (trans. by Wm. H. Woglom): *The Riddle of Cancer*, Yale Univ. Press, New Haven, 1944)

- Why does the urinary excretion of chorionic gonadotrophin fall concomitantly with the degeneration of the trophoblast?
- After more than 99 per cent of the trophoblast has been removed from the placenta, why does its size remain unaffected though its invasive and erosive properties are entirely lost?
- Why are pregnancy trophoblast cells often indistinguishable histologically from the somatic cells in the uterine wall of the pregnant host?
- Why is it that the removal of normal pregnancy trophoblast to tissue culture will result in a fiercely malignant exhibition of such trophoblast toward *all* non-trophoblast cells?

Any attempt to implement clinically the trophoblastic or unitarian thesis should be made in the light of the answers to these questions.

RADIATION

Were malignant cells actually selectively susceptible to radiations, the most malignant exhibitions of cancer would be the most amenable to therapy, since they would then contain the highest concentration of radio-sensitive cells. Chorionepithelioma and malignant melanoma represent two of the most malignant exhibitions of cancer, yet they are radio-resistant. Glioblastoma multiforme and neurogenic sarcoma are also examples of highly malignant exhibitions of cancer that are radio-resistant.

We may generalize that the malignant component of a tumor is *slightly* less radio-resistant than the somatic connective tissue stroma, but considerably more radio-resistant than the somatic parenchyma. This is why radiation often results in an increase in tumor fibrosity, which would be an excellent sign were this achieved at the cost of the radio-resistant malignant component (trophoblast) rather than at the cost of the somatic parenchyma. The so-called radio-sensitivity of a tumor is determined primarily by the radio-sensitivity of the somatic cells in which the constant malignant component happens to reside - not by the uniformly radio-resistant constant malignant component, the ectopic trophoblast.

RADIOACTIVE ELEMENTS
The most commonly used radioactive element is that of iodine in the therapy of cancer of the thyroid. Rhoads describes the limitations of this therapy as follows:

"The more malignant and destructive forms tend to pick up (radioactive iodine) to a lesser and lesser degree as the invasiveness increases."[152]

With an increase in the malignancy of the exhibition, there is necessarily an increase in the concentration of the definitively malignant cells (trophoblast) and a consequent decrease in somatic thyroid cells, which are the cells involved in the selective uptake of radioactive iodine. The decrease in tumefaction as a result of the uptake of radioactive iodine is an expression of the loss of functional somatic cells. This fact is further demonstrated in the successful use of this technique in toxic goiter.

SURGERY
The lower the concentration of trophoblast cells in a malignant lesion, the more amenable the lesion is to successful surgery. For this reason highly malignant growths like chorionepithelioma are generally inoperable.

PANCREATIC ENZYME THERAPY
The palliative use of the crystalline pancreatic enzymes in advanced human cancer rests entirely upon the validity of the unitarian or trophoblastic thesis of cancer.

CONCLUSION
Our own studies, too, appear to confirm the unitarian or trophoblastic thesis of cancer. The independently proved uniformities - which increase in degree of uniformity with the malignancy of the growth - of malignant lesions in the concentration of eight water-soluble vitamins: in vitamin C content; in water content; in cyctochrome-e; in effect on liver catalase of the host; in Warburg's criteria of glycolysis; in lactic acid formation; in

---

[152] Rhoads, C. P.: Medical Uses of Atomic Energy in U.S. and U.N. Report Series 5 - *The Int. Control of Atomic Energy*, Dept. State Publication, 2261, 1946

sugar content; in the respiratory response to added substrates; in a common means of induction; in antichymotryptic factors; in autonomy, invasiveness and erosiveness; in ability to metastasize; in amenability to universal therapeutic measures; in the general anticarcinogenic effect of caloric restriction on the incidence of mammary tumors and leukemia alike in experimental animals; in heterotransplantability; in loss of specialized function as malignancy increases (in all tumors except chorionepithelioma); in departure from the histology of the site of origin (except in primary uterine chorionepitheliomas); in numerous enzymes - all these uniformities, indeed, exclude any but an unitarian nature of cancer.[153]

Then as we examine the most malignant exhibition of cancer possible – chorionepithelioma - to find it comprised of trophoblast cells indistinguishable cytologically, endocrinologically or otherwise from those of normal pregnancy trophoblast, the fact becomes compelling that if cancer is, indeed, a unitarian phenomenon, all of its properties must be exemplified in these most primitive of all cells in the life-cycle, the trophoblast cells. These cells in their normal canalization of pregnancy (as well as *in vitro*) exhibit *every, known property of malignant* cells - though normally directed in pregnancy toward the physiological exploitation of the truly malignant process implicit in the embedding of the tissue of the conceptus into that of the mother.

Then, were all else evidential of the unitarian or trophoblastic nature of cancer set aside, and were there left for scrutiny but the

---

[153] These are, indeed, instances in which the exception proves the rule; for, were cancer not trophoblastic, its own malignant exhibition – chorionepithelioma - would then show the greatest loss of function and the greatest deviation from the histology of the site of the origin, instead of actually showing an accentuation in the normal function of trophoblast, as it does. Yet were one to attempt to ascribe to the malignant exhibition of trophoblast some intrinsic but subtle change from that of the non-malignantly exhibited trophoblast, such an attempt would be rendered nugatory by the fact that the most malignant of cancer possible in the male – chorionepithelioma - comprises trophoblast cells indistinguishable from those of pregnancy or chorionepithelioma in the female; yet, in the male, chorionepithelioma represents the widest possible deviation in histology and function from the site of origin. The latter fact corroborates the proof of a rule previously proved by its exception.

single fact that primary exhibitions of trophoblast (chorionepithelioma) are not infrequently seen that metastasize to an adenocarcinomatous or sarcomatous exhibition, and vice versa, then reason would admit of only one explanation: the trophoblastic or unitarian fact of cancer.

Were the cellular counterpart of cancer not an inextricable component of the life-cycle, represented in the most primitive cell of that cycle, the processes of natural selection themselves would have precluded the survival of the spontaneously generated cells that any alternative to the trophoblastic fact of cancer necessitates.

The unitarian thesis is not a dogma inflexibly held by its proponents; it is merely the only explanation that finds *total* congruence with all established facts on cancer. While the unitarian or trophoblastic thesis seemingly admits of no alternative, it warrants the most corrosive scrutiny. For cancer either is or is not an unitarian phenomenon, and thereby it is either trophoblastic or not trophoblastic in nature. The definitive cancer cell is either the most primitive cell in the life-cycle or it is not the most primitive. It is either the result of the *differentiation or* meiosis (however spatially or temporally anomalous) of a cell or it is not the result of cellular differentiation. It either has its normal cellular counterpart in the life-cycle, and thus is the result of cellular differentiation; or it has no cellular counterpart in the life-cycle, does not arise through cellular differentiation, and, therefore, is spontaneously created. The diploid totipotent cells within the soma, like their normally canalized daughter cells, can either undergo meiosis and subsequent trophoblast production, in response to sufficient organizer stimuli, or they can not. The occurrence of frank trophoblast cells within the soma *(invariably* as the most malignant exhibition of cancer) is either the result of the meiosis of a diploid totipotent cell or it is not; and, therefore, is the result of a spontaneous generation. The trophoblast or the cancer cell either produces specific inhibitors to pancreatic chymotrypsin and trypsin, or it does not (and the twenty or so independent workers who have so reported are all in error). A malignant tumor is either a composite tissue or it is not a composite tissue. The malignancy of a tumor is either determined by the concentration of a constant malignant component; or it is not so determined and depends, therefore, upon the successive spontaneous generation of a series of specific cells to account for the increasing malignant evolution of the tumor.

The trophoblastic or unitarian thesis holds the affirmative of all these propositions. It holds that any alternative to them will result in a *reductio ad absurdum*. The unitarian thesis recognizes the need for an orderly defined common ground of theory upon which all workers in cancer may at least meet, if not agree. It holds as reasonable the thesis that the more tenable of *two distinctly opposed hypotheses* should be given the greater credence in determining the direction of future research. It holds that in the intensive study of the peculiar metabolism of trophoblast both in pure cultures and *in vivo,* with the goal of the selective lysis of the trophoblast cell or the occlusion of its metabolism, the cancer problem may find practical resolution. It holds that the cancer problem need not offer amnesty to unbridled empiricism and negation to the most basic tenets of the rational process.

Above all else, the trophoblastic or unitarian thesis urges that the alternative non-trophoblastic or non-unitarian thesis, which is at present overwhelmingly the dominant hypothesis, be scrutinized in the light of whatever experimental evidence might exist in its support.[154] Indeed, the evaluation of any alternative to the trophoblastic or unitarian thesis - within the context of experimental facts and scientific logic - by those who find the trophoblastic or unitarian thesis untenable or tenuous, should prove most instructive. For in cancer, as in all else, facts do not speak for themselves but must be spoken for.

---

[154] In reviewing over 17,000 papers on cancer and related biological subjects, the senior author of this report, in the course of his text on "The Biological Basis of Cancer", has not found a single valid contribution that fails to find congruence with, and illumination from the trophoblastic or unitarian thesis of cancer.

NITRILOSIDES (LAETRILES) - THEIR RATIONALE AND CLINICAL UTILIZATION IN HUMAN CANCER

Ernst T. Krebs Jr. and N. R. Bouzaine MD, Ph.D

INTRODUCTION

Some twenty years of research by Ernst T. Krebs, Jr. and associates of the John Beard Memorial Foundation in California, have confirmed the suggestion of John Beard of Edinburgh University sixty years ago that the primitive trophoblast cell is the constant malignant component of all exhibitions of cancer. At least one chemical produced by this cell, human chorionic gonadotrophic hormone (hCGH), permits detection of cancer at a very early stage.

We have been using non-toxic nitrilosides (Laetrile), to which the trophoblast is susceptible, on terminal cancer cases for more than three years in Canada under the sponsorship of The McNaughton Foundation. Obviously, the nitrilosides (Laetriles) would be better used prophylactically or therapeutically at a much earlier stage in the disease.

The results of this clinical evaluation will be presented following an outline of the scientific basis of this approach.

SCIENTIFIC BASIS OF THIS THERAPY

Effective, rational chemotherapy in human cancer depends ultimately upon whether this is biologically and biochemically a single disease or a multiplicity of diseases. As proponents of the Unitarian or Trophoblastic Thesis of Cancer, we believe that all established evidence supports the former.[155] We maintain that the trophoblast cell is the constant malignant component not only of the malignant exhibition of cancer, chorionepithelioma, but also of all other exhibitions of cancer howsoever morphologically masked; and that it is in every way identical with normal pregnancy trophoblast.

It is another tenet of Beardianism that, just as the trophoblast of pregnancy is held in check first by the normally functioning maternal pancreas alone, and later by the fetal pancreas as well, the malignant induction of ectopic trophoblast likewise is prevented by

---

[155] Krebs, E.T., Jr., E.T. Krebs, Sr., and H.H. Beard, "The Unitarian or Trophoblastic Thesis of Cancer," *Medical Record*, 163:- 149-174 (1950)

the enzymatic processes of an intact pancreas. Should there be a deficiency however of pancreatic enzymes (be it of genetic, infectious, degenerative, etc., origin) the uninhibited overgrowth of the placental of ectopic trophoblast results in a hydatidiform mole or a chorionepithelioma, or in an exhibition of malignancy at the ectopic site, as the case may be.

From theoretical consideration, then, the use of modified, more sensitive, micro-Aschheim Zondek tests[156] should demonstrate the presence of chorionic gonadotrophin[157] in the blood and urine of patients with chorionepitheliomas and much lower concentrations of this same cytotrophoblastic hormone in all other exhibitions of cancer - the concentration being proportional to the biological level of malignancy.[158] These micro-Aschheim Zondek tests can also be used to evaluate the response of all types of cancer to chemotherapeutic agents.

Roffo's laboratory, Howard Beard, and Navarro and his colleagues at the University of Santo Thomas and the municipal of Manila have all reported positive curacy in large series of cancer and non-cancer patients respectively. They have all reported instances of subclinical detection of cancer or its recurrence prior to biopsy, cytology study or Roentragram. Clinical investigators with Laetrile have reported cases in which consistently positive HCGH tests have become negative after parenteral administration. The amelioration of non-specific signs and symptoms associated with positive reactors has accompanied many such instances.

---

[156] Terrel, T.C., and H.H. Beard, "A Biochemical Test for Chorionic Gonadotrophin in the Urine and Its Value as an Aid in the Diagnosis of Pregnancy and Malignancy," *South. M. J.* 48:1352-1360 (1955); Navarro, M.D., "Early Cancer Detection," *J. Philippine M.A.*, 36:425-432 (1959)

[157] Velardo, J.T., *The Anatomy and Endocrine Physiology of the Female Reproductive System, in the Endochinology of Reproduction* (J.T. Velardo, Ed.), New York, Oxford University Press, 1958, p.189; Kupperman, H.S., and J.A. Epstein, *Hormone Changes in Pregnancy, in Essentials of Human Reproduction* (J.T. Velardo, Ed.), New York, Oxford University Press, 1958, p. 91

[158] Ferguson, *J.A.M.A.*, 101:1933 (1933), cited in Boyd, W., A Text-Book of Pathology, Philadelphia, Lea and Febiger, ed. 4, 1943, p. 642

BETA-GLUCURONIDASE

Independent of the foregoing considerations, Fishman in 1947 reported the presence of B-glucuronidase in malignant tissue.[159] This enzyme, which hydrolyses B-glucuronoside after the latter has been produced by oxidation of B-glucoside, was first reported to exist in animal tissue by Sera in 1914.[160] Fishman and Anlyan have described levels of B-glucuronidase in surgically removed specimens of cancers of the breast, uterus, stomach and mesentary, abdominal wall, and esophagus 100 to 3600 times as high as levels of this enzyme in corresponding uninvolved tissue.[161] While they have empirically interpreted this as "a metabolic response of the tissue to estrogen or a related substance", Beardianism maintains that this is directly related to the fact that the syncytial trophoblast produces abundant quantities of estrogenic and related steroids.[162] These steroids elicit from the hostal tissue the production of B-glucuronidase necessary for their detoxification as the corresponding B-steroid glycuronosides, which are ultimately excreted in the urine as physiologically inert.

RHODANESE

In addition to their high levels of B-glucuronidase, malignant lesions are characterized by a generally profound deficiency of most other enzymes and a specific deficiency in rhodanese as was

---

[159] Fishman, W.H., "B-Glucuronidase Activity of Blood and Tissue of Obstetrical and Surgical Patients," *Science*, 105:646 (1947)

[160] Sera, Y., "Aur Kenntnis der Gepaarten Glukuronsaure, 111 Ueber die Spaltung der Orcin - und Chloroglucinglukuronsaure durch Organsafte," *Z. Physiol. Chem.* 92:261-275 (1914)

[161] Fishman, W.H., and A.J. Anlyan, "A Comparison of the 13-Glucuronidase Activity of Normal, Tumor, and Lymph Node Tissues of Surgical Patients," *Science*, 106:66-67 (1947); Fishman, W.H., and A.J. Anlyan, "The Presence of High B-Glucuronidase Activity in Cancer Tissue," *J. Biol. Chem.*, 169: 449-450 (1947); Fishman, W.H., and A.J. Anlyan, "B-Glucuronidase Activity in Human Tissues. Some Correlations with the Processes of Malignant Growth and with the Physiology of Reproduction," Fourth Intl. .Cancer Research Congress, 6:1034-1041 (1950)

[162] Beard, J., "The Embryology of Tumors," *Anat. Anz.*, 486-494 (1903); *Centrbl. L.allig. Path. Anat.*, 14:513-520, (1903); Beard, J., "The Interlude of Cancer," *Med. Record*, 69:1020 (1903)

reported by Homburger and Mendel, Rodney and Bowman.[163] Rosenthal reported an 80% decrease in rhodanese in hepatomatous liver tissue, and a similar decrease was found in the leukemic invasion of tissues.[164]

Lang, who discovered this enzyme in 1933, found that it converts hydrocyanic acid to rhodanate (thiocyanate or sulfocyanate) in the presence of thiosulfate or colloid sulfur thusly:[165]

HCN + Na₂S₂O₃-----------------Na SCN+NaHSO₃

Sumner and Somers point out that rhodanese undoubtedly prevents the accumulation of excessively toxic exhibitions of HCN arising from the scission of dietary *B*-glycuronosides and *B*-glucosides by paralleling them both in sites of occurrence and in concentration.[166] It exceeds the concentration of *B*-glucuronidase and *B*-glucosidase in all but malignant tissues. Whether or not human chorionic gonadotrophin produced by exhibitions of lesser malignancy accounts for the absence of rhodanese in the definitely malignant (trophoblast) cells, the fact that it does account for such rhodanese deficiency in the immediately contiguous somatic cells was demonstrated by Sanchez and Bertran.[167] They reported that five international units of an aqueous solution of chorionic gonadotrophin 24 hours after injection decreased rhodanese activity in the tissue of rats 90% or more.

---

[163] Homburger, I., and Fishman, W,H., The Physiopathology of Cancer, New York, Patil B. Hoeber, Inc., 1955, p. 842; Mendel, B., H. Rodney and M.C. Bowman, "Rhodanese and the Pasteur Effect," *Cancer Research*, 6:45 (1946)

[164] Giordano,.G., A. Violante, G. Lerenzetti, and U. Sapio, "Rhodanese Activity of the Neoplastic and Hemopoietic Tissue of Rats with Myeloma in Leukemic Phase," *Biochemie. Appl.* 3:284 (1956)

[165] Lang, K., "Die Rhodanbildung im Tierkooper," *Biochem. Z.*, 259:243-256 (1933); cf, Lang, K., *Z.Vitamin-hormonu-Ferment-Forsch.*, 2:288-291 (1949) (a review)

[166] Summer, J.B., and G.F. Somers, Chemistry and Methods of Enzymes, New York, Academic Press, 1947, p. 98

[167] Sanchez, F., and E. Castella Bertran, "Variations in the Rhodanese Activity Induced by Injection of Chorionic Gonadotrophin," *An. Facul. Vet. Univ. Madrid y Inst Invest. Vet.*, 3:78-82 (1951) (English summary)

CYANOPHORIC GLUCOSIDES AND CYANOPHORIC GLUCURONOSIDES

Aware of the high concentration of B-glucuronidase in malignant tissue, Danielli in 1950[168], and Conchie, Hay, and Levy[169], and Williams[170] in 1961 suggested the use of glucuronides as tumor-inhibiting agents. Working within the context of the unitarian or trophoblastic thesis of cancer, Krebs and others, as early as 1925 observed in crude vegetable extracts definitive palliative and therapeutic properties with respect to human cancer.[171] In the 1940's he identified this property with such constituents of B-cyanogenetic glucosides as prunasin (l-mandelonitrile-B-glucoside) and amygdalin (d,l-gentio-bioside). These materials were isolated in crystalline form and demonstrated to be non-toxic. Subsequent synthesis of specific glycuronosides such as 1-mandelonitrile-B-glycuronoside has provided preparations with therapeutic properties substantially superior to the previously demonstrated activity of the glucosidic nitrilosides.[172] A large homologous series of nitrilosides with widely varying aglycones and sugars is now under study.

PHARMACOLOGY AND TOXICOLOGY

When the Laetriles are incubated *in vitro* with a B-glucosidase, there is a quantitative and dramatic release of HCN, nascent above its boiling point of 26°C. McIlroy,[173] and Edmunds and Gunn[174]

---

[168] Danielli, J.F., "Cell Physiology and Pharmacology," London, Eisevier Publishing Co., 1950

[169] Conchie, J., A.J. Hay, and G.A. Levy, "Mammalian Glycosidases," *J. Biochem.,* 79:324 (May, 1961)

[170] Williams, R.T., "Detoxication Mechanisms and the Design of Drugs, in Biological Approaches to Cancer Chemotherapy" (R. J.C. Harris, Ed.), London and New York, Academic Press, 1961, p. 36

[171] Lowman, A., "Carbohydrate Metabolism and Its Relation to the Cancer Problem," Doctoral Thesis in Pharmacology, University of California, 1939

[172] Guidetti, E., "Preliminary Observations on Some Cases of Cancer Treated by Cyanogenetic Glucuronoside," Acta Union Internationale Contretre Le Cancer, 11:156-158 (1955), "Osservazioni Cliniche Sugli Effetti-therapeutici di un Glycuronoside Cianogenetico in Casi di Neoplasie Maligne Umane," *Gazzetta Medica Italiana,* 1-19 (1958)

[173] McIlroy, R. J., *The Plant Glycosides*, London, Edward Arnold and Co., 1951, p.9-10

have demonstrated a clear counterpart to this reaction in both plants and animals.

The Laetriles are hydrolyzed *in vivo* to free nascent HCN, benzaldehyde, and a sugar or its acid. As previously explained, the HCN is detoxified in somatic tissue by rhodanese to thiocyanate, which is then eliminated in the saliva, sweat, bile, and urine. The benzaldehyde is immediately oxidized to benzoic acid and detoxified through the liver by glycine conjugation as hippuric acid and/or glucuronic acid conjugation as benzoyl glycuronoside.

Since these nitrilosides are reasonably homologous with natural compounds found in many edible plants, and since all detoxification products are normal constituents of human blood and urine, they are expectedly free of toxicity. The intact Laetrile molecule is devoid of pharmacological or toxicological properties, these being present only after hydrolysis. Although free HCN is very volatile and may be lethal on inhalation, the cyanogenetic glycuronosides are non-toxic when administered parenterally. One gram of d,l-mandelonitrile-*B*-glycuronoside contains 30 mg of incipient HCN, and doses of over 5 grams have been administered intravenously without toxic effects. In normal tissues the excess of rhodanese, as compared with *B*-glucosidase and *B*-glucuronidase, results in the detoxification of scission products; but as the result of the lack of rhodanese in malignant cells, the HCN released by *B*-glucuronidase is not detoxified and remains free to exert its lethal effects against such cells and the contiguous somatic in which rhodanese is inhibited by chorionic gonadotrophin. Stern and Willheim, in their "Biochemistry of Malignant Tumors", have summarized evidence for the selective sensitivity of cancer cells to cyanides.[175]

The present Laetriles depend for their cancericidal action almost exclusively upon potential HCN, although Waterman has reported that benzaldehyde impedes the growth of inoculated tumors when

---

[174] Edmunds, C. W., and J. A. Gunn, *Cushnys Pharmacology and Therapeutics* (ed. 12), Philadelphia, Lea and Febiger, 1940, pp. 682-685
[175] Stern, K. and R. Wilheim, *The Biochemistry of Malignant Tumors*, Brooklyn, New York, Reference Press, 1943

brought into direct contact with the inoculum.[176] Utilization of cancericidal aglycones and sugar derivatives will, of course, augment the present cancericidal action. While benzaldehyde and benzoic acid are, for example, antiseptic as well as analgesic, the substitution of an hydroxyl radical in the benzaldehyde ring would of course yield a more active analgesic upon hydrolysis - salicylic acid.

CLINICAL EVALUATION OF LAETRILE

Every chemical, reaction, product of reaction, source of reactant, and means of detoxification described above has been independently established and generally accepted. However, although the high concentration of B-glucuronidase, the apparent presence of a source of estrogen, and the deficiency of rhodanese have been empirically established in all exhibitions of cancer, acceptance of the above explanation of these phenomena in malignancies other than chorionepitheliomas is limited to adherents of the unitarian or trophoblastic thesis of cancer. We therefore feel that the Laetriles should be treated empirically as isolates in terms of ordinary clinical practicability until proof of their utility and acceptance of that proof permits their return to this unified context of Beardianism.

The purpose of this clinical investigation was to determine whether there could be obtained at the malignant focus, a release of HCN of a magnitude sufficient to yield a substantial cytotoxic effect without exposing the host to undue toxicity. With the assistance of several medical associates, a wide variety of terminal cancer cases, on whom all conventional methods of treatment had previously proved unsuccessful or inadvisable, were selected.

ADMINISTRATION

Laetrile is soluble in distilled water or normal salt solution and is administered parenterally. While some clinical investigators have given it intramuscularly, intrapleurally, intraperitoneally, locally, by means of arterial perfusion, and by iontophoresis, we have thus far confined our work to the intravenous and intramuscular, as well

---

[176]   Waterman, N., "Der Heutige Stand Der Chemotherapeutischen Carcinoforschung," *Ergebn. der inn.med u Kinderk.* 30:304- 376. (1946)

as administration by high retention enema and injection directly into certain lesions. Primary and secondary carcinomas of the lung have proved to be the most amenable to this route of therapy, because it avoids the rich reservoirs of B-glucuronidase in the liver, spleen, and kidneys. The most desirable route in malignancies beyond these organs can only be determined by an intelligent consideration of such factors as the underlying anatomy and physiopathology, the extent of the metastases, and the concentration of B-glucuronidase in the cells.

There has been considerable variation in the dosage of Laetrile administered. In the early 1950's Navarro and others used 50-100 mg doses and in 1957 these were increased to 250-500 mg.[177] The total dosage a patient received seldom exceeded 2 grams. We feel now that each patient should receive a minimum of 30 grams. In some cancers, such as carcinoma of the breast, and in instances when only a brief stay in hospital was possible, Laetrile was given in doses of 3 grams per day for 10 successive days. Other doctors have preferred to give 1 gram per day for 30 days.

It is our conclusion that, where time permits, it is most desirable to give the patient 1 gram of Laetrile every second day for the first 1-2 weeks. When it becomes evident that the drug is effective and that the patient is able to tolerate the breakdown of malignant tissue, this should be increased to 1 gm per day until the minimum dosage of 30 grams is attained. Such a routine produces results which are equally as good as those obtained with larger doses and seems to offer the advantage of taxing the regenerative processes of the body less severely.

In a few of the most terminal and hopeless cases, death ensued before adequate treatment could be given. But many of the patients, having received the basic 30 grams of Laetrile and having then continued on a maintenance dosage of 1-2 grams per week, became ambulatory and gradually resumed their normal activities.

---

[177] Navarro Manuel D., "Laetrile Therapy in Cancer," read at Eighth International Cancer Congress, Moscow, Russia, July 22-28, 1962. Reprinted in The Philippine Journal of Cancer, July-Sept., 1962

SUPPLEMENTARY THERAPY

It has been our experience that, while Laetrile alone has proved to be effective, even better results can be obtained with some supplementary therapy as well. Pangamic acid (Vitamin B15) is a methylating agent which appears to improve liver function with respect to its capacity to detoxify elements released from the malignant lesion following Laetrile therapy. Our patients received 100-200 mg of pangamic acid intramuscularly daily during their stay in hospital. Thereafter, a similar dosage was given with each maintenance dose of Laetrile. This substance may also be given orally should the patient so request it; but it appears to be more effective when given intramuscularly.

CRITERIA FOR EVALUATION

The progress of our patients was measured by a consideration of the clinical signs and symptoms, and by pathological, cytological, and radiological reports. Samples of the blood and urine were analyzed at intervals to detect any alterations in hematopoietic processes or in renal function during treatment.

RESULTS

Of the cases treated, the results serve to illustrate the wide range of malignancies which respond to Laetrile therapy. It is hoped that the following cases might further illustrate our conclusions.

CASE #1

Mr. A.G., 44-year-old radio announcer, was perfectly well until May 1960. When examined on June 7th he complained of disphagia and otalgia of one-month duration. Examination revealed a left anterior tonsillar pillar which was indurated, Leukoplastic, and thickened at its inferior insertion. There was no evidence of adenopathy. A diagnosis of epidermoid carcinoma (Grade 1) was made on the basis of histopathological report following biopsy. Because of the radio-resistance of such lesions, the radiotherapy which had been initiated was discontinued and the patient was submitted to cobalt therapy during June, July and August. The lesion continued to progress and his general condition worsened; but, because of his occupation, he refused surgery. By March 20, 1961, cervical brachial, and coronary adenopathy had developed to the extent that surgery was impossible. He had been able to swallow only liquids for six months.

On March 23, 1961, Laetrile therapy (1 gram per day I.V.) plus B15 (100 mg per day I.M.) was begun. After the first 6 grams of Laetrile progression of the lesion was halted and by April 4th he was released from hospital in a much improved condition. Dosage was reduced to 1 gram of Laetrile and 100mg of B15 twice per week. By June 27, 1961, the dysphagia, adenopathy, and otalgia had disappeared, the primary lesion was considerably reduced in size, and the patient had gained 11 pounds.

During the last year, on a regimen of 1 gram Laetrile and 100 mgs of B15 one to two times per week, his condition has continued to improve and there is no longer any evidence of the primary lesion. With cessation of treatment with Laetrile for more than 6 weeks the dysphagia and otalgia return but there has been no recurrence of the primary lesion or of the cervical adenopathy. The patient should therefore continue on maintenance dosage indefinitely.

CASE #2:

Mrs. G.S., 63-year-old housewife, was first diagnosed as having a glandular epithelioma of the left breast with metastases in Nov. 1959. A radical mastectomy was performed at that time, and from Jan. 22 to April 4, 1960, she received radiotherapy (13,230 r to the left exillary and supraclavicular regions, left chest, and mediastinum) on May 5, 1961, she was admitted to hospital completely incapacitated by pain and by intense dyspnea and severe coughing at the least effort. Physical and radiological examination revealed metastases to the right and left supraclavicular nodes and to both lungs - probably due to radiotherapy. Cytology reports on a left pleural effusion were negative. During her stay in hospital she received 200 mg of B15 intramuscularly each day and 1 gm of Laetrile intravenously every second day from May 24th until July 21st. From July 21st to July 28th she received 3 gms of Laetrile per day. Within a month after Laetrile therapy was begun her dyspnea and cough had disappeared and she had become ambulatory. When released from hospital on July 28, 1961, the patient appeared clinically to be greatly improved, although X-ray studies of the lungs showed no change with the exception of the absence of any pleural effusion.

Since that time she continued to receive 1 gram of Laetrile I.V. and 200 mg of B 15 I.M. twice weekly. Her pain almost completely disappeared, she is no longer troubled by dyspnea or coughing, and she gradually resumed her normal activities. It can be seen that her blood picture improved and there has been no evidence of any toxicity.

CASE #3:
Mrs. L.N., 52 year old housewife, was admitted to hospital March 6, 1962, with complaints of metrorrhagia of three months' duration (menopause 6 years ago) and of right upper quadrant pain and dyspepsia of fifteen days' duration. On the basis of clinical evidence and the cytological report following curettage, a diagnosis of adenocarcinoma of the uterus (class V) was made. The patient was started on Laetrile on March 21, 1962, receiving intravenously 1 gm per day for three days and then 500 mg every second day, until her release from hospital on May 22nd. She was also given 100 mg of B15 every other day during hospitalization. A second cytological report on April 26th revealed no evidence of adenocarcinoma but only of endocervical hyperplasia. Her abdominal pain and metrorrhagia had ceased by this time and she had begun to gain weight. Since her release from hospital we have continued to give her 1 gm of Laetrile I.V. and 100 mg of B15 I.M. twice weekly. She has had no recurrence of symptoms, has regained her appetite and strength, is sleeping better, and does her housework without effort. Her urine, which originally contained traces of albumin and bacteria, mucus, hyalin casts and calcium oxylate crystals, is now normal. Her blood picture has not changed significantly, although Vita-Iron has been used to maintain her hemoglobin levels. No toxicity has been noted.

CASE #4:
This 55-year-old patient, Mr. G.G., was admitted to hospital June 2, 1962. A barium series and cineflurography at another hospital on May 7, 1962 had revealed an epithelioma of the esophagus. There was evidence of mucosal ulceration and of severe narrowing of the lumen for a length of 10 cm at the junction of the middle and lower

thirds of the esophagus. At the time of admission to this hospital he was near death - unable to take any solid food and, in fact, even regurgitating liquids. He complained of pain in the right upper quadrant. X-rays of the lungs on June 4th revealed an ill-defined opacity in the right middle lobe suggestive of pneumonia (he had been treated with tetracycline 2 weeks before for pneumonia), and pleural thickening and effusion on the left side. It was uncertain whether left pulmonary metastases were present.

The patient was treated with Fortemycin and with 1 gram of Laetrile I.V. and 100 mg of B15 I.M. daily. He required Phenergan and Demerol in order to sleep at night. His pain fever had disappeared within 6 days, and after two weeks in hospital he was able to eat solid foods, had gained twelve pounds, and was ambulatory. X-rays of the lungs on June 16th were normal with exception of some pleural thickening in the left axillary line. On June 24, 1962, the patient was released from hospital. Treatment was reduced to 1 gram of Laetrile I.V. and 100 mg of B15 I.M. every second day. X-ray studies of the lungs on July 27th were normal. A barium meal at this time revealed that the mucosa of an 8 cm segment of the distal third of the esophagus was irregular and that the lumen was somewhat reduced in caliber, but that the barium passed through without obstruction. The patient at present feels well and has returned to work. He no longer requires analgesics to sleep. His urine has been normal throughout the course of treatment; but his hematocrit and hemoglobin, which were 31% and 10.2 gm% respectively on June 4th had increased to 37% and 11.8 gm% respectively by July 7th. There has been no evidence of toxicity.

CASE #5:
Mrs. G.M., 53 years old, was first discovered to have a glandular epithelioma of the ascending colon on August 20, 1961, at which time a resection and anastamosis was done. On February 15, 1962, she presented with symptoms of obstruction. This was confirmed by barium enema and a second operation was performed on Feb. 20th. A recurrence of the glandular epithelioma was found at the site of anastomosis; this had spread to involve the posterior abdominal wall, a number of mesenteric lymph nodes, and the greater omentum. It was impossible to excise the entire mass, but a

side to side anastomosis of the terminal part of the ileum and the transverse colon was performed to relieve the obstruction.

She was then started on Laetrile, receiving 500 mg I.V. every second day for six days, then 1 gm per day for another six days. She has received 1 gm of Laetrile every second day since that time, and has also been given 200 mg of B15 I.M. with each injection of Laetrile. At present she is feeling very well and is able to perform her household duties without difficulty. Her pain and colic is greatly diminished, her appetite has improved, her bowels are functioning normally, and she has no difficulty sleeping. There has been a noticeable reduction in the size of her abdominal mass. Urinalyses have remained normal and her hemoglobin, which had dropped to 10.6 gm% following her operation in February, has increased to 11.7 gm%. There has been no indication of any toxicity.

CONCLUSION
To maintain that any of these patients has been cured – "cure" being defined as a five-year period free of tumor recurrence - is not our purpose. In accordance with the concepts of Beardianism, cancer, like pellagra or scurvy, is a deficiency disease which must be controlled either permanently or until the enzymatic deficiency of the pancreas is rectified. It appears to us that the effectiveness of the Laetrile as much a palliative has been clearly demonstrated in a wide variety of malignant exhibitions, particularly in primary and secondary neoplasms of the lung.

It is also very evident that Laetrile possesses strong analgesic properties; and, although none of the patients mentioned in the above reports were troubled with fetor, in other cases treated, this symptom was also relieved when present. Furthermore, there has been no indication of any toxicity in any of our cases, in spite of the large amounts of Laetrile administered. In view of these facts it would seem only reasonable to suggest that this drug be more properly evaluated prior to the use of other palliatives, immediately following the detection of cancer.

It should be remembered too that to date the successful resolution of the anemias, vitamin deficiencies, and all other chronic diseases has only been accomplished by non-toxic physiologic means of prophylactic significance. Whether the systemically non-toxic and apparently cancericidal Laetriles are also of preventative as well as palliative import is certainly worthy of additional scrutiny.

SUMMARY
1. Malignant tumors are focally characterized by a high concentration of B-glucuronidase and a deficiency of rhodanese.
2. Specific nitrilosides (Laetriles), which upon hydrolysis yield hydrogen cyanide, an aglycone (benzaldehyde) and a sugar moiety, have been prepared to exploit this B-glucuronidase-rhodanese pattern.
3. Following parenteral administration, there appears to be released in a wide variety of selectively sensitive malignant tissues such an excess of nascent HCN as to produce effects of definite palliative, and possible prophylactic, consequences in human cancer.
4. Laetrile also possesses strong analgesic properties and shows no evidence of any toxicity.
5. On the basis of the results reported in this paper and those obtained by other clinical investigators using Laetrile, it is suggested that this drug might be more properly evaluated in less terminal cases untreated by other palliatives.

LAETRILE THERAPY IN CANCER

Manuel D. Navarro, M.D.
Associate Professor, Faculty of Medicine & Surgery, University of
Santo Tomas, Manila, Philippines

Read at the 8th International Cancer Congress, Moscow. July 22-28, 1962.
Reprinted from *The Philippine Journal of Cancer,* July-Sept., 1962

About the author: Dr Manuel Navarro, former Professor of Medicine 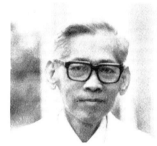 and Surgery at the University of Santo Tomas, Manila. Associate Member of the National Research Council of the Philippines. A Fellow of the Philippine College of Physicians, the Philippine Society of Endocrinology and Metabolism. A member of the Philippine Medical Association, the Philippine Cancer Society and many other medical groups. Dr Navarro is an internationally recognised cancer researcher with over 100 major scientific papers to his credit, some read before the International Cancer Congress. Dr Navarro has treated terminally ill cancer patients with Laetrile for over 25 years. He stated in the *Cancer News Journal*: *"It is my carefully considered clinical judgement, as a practising oncologist and researcher in this field, that I have obtained most significant and encouraging results with the use of Laetrile-amygdalin in the treatment of terminal cancer patients..."*
[178]

---

[178] *Cancer News Journal,* Jan/April 1971, pp.19-21

Since the last report on Laetrile (nitriloside) therapy for advanced cancer at the International Union Against Cancer Symposium on Cancer Chemotherapy for the Pacific-Asian Area in Tokyo in 1957, the dosage of Laetrile (nitriloside) has been considerably increased.[179] In 1953 it ranged from 50-100 mg; in 1957, 250-500 mg and the most the writer gave to patients who have benefited from the drug was a little over 2 grains. Now, the dose ranges from 1,000 to 2,000 mg intravenously daily and as much as 3,000 mg for a minimum total of 30 grams a dose is considerably greater than the writer or the others have used in 1952.

It would seem that there is some degree of parallelism between penicillin and Laetrile (nitriloside) as regards dosage. When the former was found excellent for several infections caused by Gram-positive or Gram-negative microorganisms, it was reportedly a failure in sub-acute bacterial endocarditis at the routine dose of 100,000 Units, until a Brooklyn physician thought of administering ten times this amount.[180] True enough, the 1,000,000 Units of penicillin proved effective in sub-acute bacterial endocarditis with the subsequent saving of thousands of patients destined to die from this disease. That the same experience on an increase of the dose for the maligned Laetrile (nitriloside) for cancer therapy holds true is borne out by the work of the Canadian investigators, pioneers in the use of the massive dosages of this drug.[181] It is very fortunate that the Beardian scientists can exchange data for each benefit from the findings of the others.

Since the mechanism of the action of Laetrile (nitriloside) is one of the ways of understanding the claims for the effectiveness of this

---

[179] Manuel Navarro, M. D.: Five Years' Experience with Laetrile Therapy in Advanced Cancer; *Philippine J. Cancer* 1:289-307 (Oct - Dec) 1957; ACTA, Vols. XV bis No.1.209-221, 1959

[180] Fishbein, M.: Personal Communication (University of Santo Tomas Conference, 1961)

[181] McNaughton Foundation Investigators: Unpublished report (personal communication)

drug in cancer, a cure for which is so desperately needed and for which the world is spending hundreds of millions of dollars, let us discuss this mechanism briefly.

The antiblastic action of Laetrile (nitriloside)[182] depends upon the scission of the molecule to a molecule of hydrocyanic acid, benzaldehyde and a sugar or its acid through the hydrolytic action of beta-glucosidase and/or beta-glucuronidase (BG).[183] The specificity of BG for the natural nitrilosides (Laetriles) or beta-cyanophoric glucosides and glycuronosides or the synthetic Laetriles (nitrilosides) has been proven *in vitro* and *in vivo*. To understand the hydrolytic action produced, one must recall the physiology of BG, which is tied to the Beardian thesis of cancer.

BG is found normally in the liver, spleen, kidneys, and to a certain extent in the leucocytes. It has the function of conjugating the estrogen with glucuronic acid to form estrogen-glycuronoside, which compound is excreted in the urine. BG is therefore responsible for the metabolic conjugation of any excess of estrogen-like steroids present in the body.

Since Cori[184] reported in 1927 on the presence of large amounts of estrogen-like steroids in cancer, other investigators have confirmed his findings.[185] Such excess formation of estrogen-like steroids in cancer therefore brings into play the physiological role of BG to

---

[182] A nitriloside or Laetrile is any cyanophoric glucoside and/or glycuronoside that, when exposed to beta-glucosidase and/or beta-glucuronidase (BG), is hydrolyzed to an aglycone, nascent hydrogen cyanide, and a sugar or its acid.

[183] BG refers to the complex of beta-glucosidases, beta-glucuronidases and other enzymes generically comprising the beta-glucuronidase focally characterizing a malignant lesion.

[184] Cori, C. E.: The Influence of Ovariectomy on the Spontaneous Occurrence of Mammary Carcinoma in Mice. *J. Exper. Med.* 45:983, 1927

[185] Dingmanse, E.; Freud, J.; de Jongh, S. E. and Laqueur, F.: Ueber das Vorkommen von Hohen Mengen Weiblichen (Sexual) Hormones Menformon in Blut von Krebskranken (Manner). *Arch. f. Gynek.*, 14 1, 225, 1930; Lewis, D. and Geschickter, C. F.: Estrin in high concentration yield by a fibroadenoma of the breast; *J. Am. Med. Assn.*: 103:646-647, 1947; Smith, O. and Emerson, K., Jr.: Urinary estrogens and related compounds in post-menopausal women with mammary cancer. Effect of Cortisone treatment. Proc. SOC. *Exper. Biol & Med.* 18:264, 1954

serve as the catalyzer for this defense mechanism. Consequently, the body causes the area where the excessive steroid formation occurs to be surrounded by a sea of BG. Such presence of a high titer of BG in cancer tissues is supported by the observations of several investigators, foremost of whom are Fishman and Anlyan.[186]

Such defense action of surrounding the cancer cell with a sea of BG is responsible for the specific action of Laetrile (nitriloside). Parenteral administration of the drug results in the hydrolysis of the Laetrile (nitriloside) molecule (laevo-mandelonitrile glycuronoside) at the cancer site by BG into HCN, benzaldehyde, glucose and/or glucuronic acid.

HCN being nascent above 26°C. will, upon its release from the Laetrile (nitriloside) molecule, diffuse into the cancer cells, causing their death; while the normal body cells adjacent to the cancer cells would not succumb to the lethal effect of the hydrocyanic acid because of the presence of rhodanese - absent or deficient in the cancer cells - which converts the poison into thiocyanate, a compound with hypotensive action. The writer has noted this hypotensive action following Laetrile (nitriloside) injections in several cancer patients suffering at the same time from hypertension.

One distinct advantage of this drug over all other anti-cancer drugs currently under investigation is that it does not depress the bone marrow and can therefore be administered for quite a long period of time.

Several cases of early cancer given this form of therapy are still alive for as long as 74 months, while the survival of the far advanced cases has been increased significantly as compared with the

---

[186] Fishman, W. H. and Anlyan, A. J.: The Presence of High Beta-glucuronidase Activity in Cancer Tissue. *J. Biol. Chem.* 169:449-450, 1947; Odel, L. D.; Burth, J. R.: B.G. activity in human female genital cancer. *Cancer Res.* 9.362-364, 1949; Campbell, J. D.: The Intracellular localization of B.G. *Brit. J. Exper. Path.*, 30:548-554, 1949; Seligman, A. M.; Maclos, M. M.; Manheimer, L. H.; Friedman, O. M. and Wolf, G.: Development of New Methods for the Histochemical Demonstration of hydrolytic Intracellular Enzymes in a Program of Cancer Research. *Ann. Surg.* 130:333-34 1, 1949

controls which did not receive Laetrile (nitriloside). One of the means of knowing when to stop or resume this form of therapy used by all Beardian scientists is the Beard Anthrone test (BAT), a modification of which was presented at the last cancer congress held in London in 1958. Several of the illustrative cases using the different doses that went hand-in-hand with the development of Laetrile (nitriloside) therapy are described below:

ILLUSTRATIVE CASES
A. 100 mg dose:
Case 9: A.G., 78, widow, underwent a simple mastectomy for a mass in the left breast that was benign to needle biopsy. The histological section, however, revealed adenocarcinoma. The BAT was ++. Two months after the operation the patient noted lymphadenopathy in the axilla with concomitant pain, itchiness and redness over the mastectomy scar. The BAT was still positive. On March 14, 1956 she was injected Laetrile (nitriloside) (100 mg) every four days for eighteen doses. Beta-glucosidase was an adjuvant then. With the injections, the patient was relieved of the pain, the itchiness and redness along the scar disappeared also. After the 12th injection, Laetrile (nitriloside) was also administered by *iontophoresis* for a total of six applications over the axillary lymphadenopathy, resulting in the disappearance of the mass, leaving only a small fibrotic nodule. Up to the present - 74 months after Laetrile (nitriloside) therapy was instituted - the patient is feeling well with no recurrence of her malignant condition. The BAT is negative.

B. 250 mg dose:
Case 19: R.P., 27, single, had a +++ BAT after undergoing pan-hysterectomy. After her operation she still had hypogastric and sacrolumbar pains and melena. Because of the positive BAT, she received postoperative irradiation and later, when the urine persistently showed positive results with the BAT, Laetrile (nitriloside) (250mg) injections every four days for three months were given. The injections relieved her of the hypogastric and sacrolumbar pains. The BAT became less positive as the treatment progressed. Because she felt so well she stopped all therapy for two months but resumed her injections when the BAT was shown to be still positive. Finally, in February 1959, exactly a year after her

operation, the BAT became negative. She is healthy and strong and presently works as secretary for a commercial firm 29 months after Laetrile (nitriloside) therapy.

C. 250-500 mg dose:

Case 68: C.B., 30, female, underwent a series of nasal operations since 1955 for the chief complaint of nasal obstruction. The first four operations were found benign in character, or at least the characteristic histological picture of malignancy was not yet evident. In all she had five operations, the last one was done in December 1958 when the excised specimen was finally reported as malignant: "Transitional cell" carcinoma. The BAT was positive at this time. She underwent radiation therapy. In June 1959 she had a recurrence of the nasal obstruction and accompanied now by bulging over the right maxillary antrum. The BAT was still positive. Biopsy was done again and the report was still the same: "transitional cell" carcinoma. The patient refused further surgical treatment, but agreed to try deep X-ray therapy and Laetrile (nitriloside) injections (she started with 250 mg and then received a few 500 mg doses). The bulging on the right antral region disappeared during the course of treatment, while the pain and the nasal obstruction were relieved. The six months of relief previously obtained with surgery and radiation therapy was now stretched to 1 1/2 years by radiation and Laetrile (nitriloside) therapy. Although she was symptom-free, the BAT was still positive. In January 1961 she became aware of the presence of pea-sized nodules - one on the chest above the right breast and the other in the right axilla. These were excised. Histological examination of the excised grayish masses revealed that these were "plasmacytoma", metastatic, from the nose and maxillary antrum. The previous biopsy slides were consequently reviewed and these too were truly "plasmacytoma". No therapy was given after excision. The BAT was still positive six months after the excision and by this time pain along the left ankle was noted by the patient. Radiological examination showed a suspicious involvement of the bones.

D. 1,000 mg dose:

Case 90: C.G., 39, female, underwent radical mastectomy of the right breast in July, 1958, followed by bilateral oophorectomy in September 1958. She was symptom-free for a year. After another year her urine became positive to the BAT, but she was still symptomless. No therapy was given her. After six months she complained of backaches. Her BAT had increased to +++. Radiological examination revealed metastatic involvement of the 9th and 10th ribs. She was placed on Thio-tepa therapy, receiving more than twenty-four injections. Because she had palpitation, weakness, and feeling of faintness after every injection, therapy was discontinued. BAT was still positive. Radiological examination of the ribs did not show any change for the better. She was placed on Laetrile (nitriloside) therapy at a dose of 1,000 mg every other day. After a total of 41,000 mg, X-ray examinations showed the ribs were practically healed - the pains have gradually disappeared too. She is on a maintenance dose of 1,000 mg twice a month. Her urine is now negative with the BAT.

Case 91: A.B., 29, female, student nurse, underwent an open and close surgery for an abdominal tumor which turned out to be malignant, affecting both ovaries and involving the sigmoid. A piece of tissue was removed and this proved to be "schirrous cystadenocarcinoma". The patient underwent a course of Thio-tepa therapy for a total of 100 mg. After this treatment she still complained of pain on defecation, hypogastric pain, melena and cough; she lost five pounds. The BAT was +++. She was then started on Laetrile (nitriloside) therapy in December and by January she was back to work as operating-room nurse. For four months she had only occasional twinges of pain; she regained the weight lost and the cough has completely disappeared. The lesion (?) in the right lung noted by radiography (when patient was still coughing) cleared up three months later. She received a total of 44,000 mg. When asked to evaluate her health, she claimed that in December it was only 50% normal; five months later it was 90%. Her urine is still positive with the BAT. She is on a 1,000 mg. dose every other day. Every now and then,. she receives the Laetrile (nitriloside) intravenously.

COMMENT

Laetrile (nitriloside) at the small dose of 100 mg administered by injection and iontophoresis has been effective particularly in early cases of metastasis (axilla) from operated breast cancer. The subsequent increase in the dose to 1,000 mg intravenously has effected more dramatic therapeutic results among the advanced cases of cancer as shown in the last two cases. The writer feels that the administration of Laetrile (nitriloside) in the 3,000-5,000 dose range would produce better anti-blastic effects.

CONCLUSION
The considerable increase in the therapeutic dose of Laetrile (nitriloside) produced more dramatic anti-blastic effects as compared to those achieved with the 50 mg dose used in 1952. These illustrative cases, though few in number, are sufficient to call to the attention of previous investigators, who claimed to have found Laetrile (nitriloside) useless at the smaller dose range, suggesting that they try the drug again in the larger dose range.

CHEMOTHERAPY OF INOPERABLE CANCER

Preliminary Report of 10 Cases Treated with Laetrile
by
John A. Morrone, M.D., F.I.C.S., A.S.A.S.
Jersey City, N.J.

Attending Surgeon, Jersey City Medical Center

The hope of the future lies in the chemotherapy of cancer. In view of deep-rooted prejudice against clinical experimentation in this field, a completely objective study and report of 10 cases should be of interest.

The use of Laetrile (l-mandelonitrile-beta-glycuronoside), a beta cyanogenetic glucoside, is based on the unitarian or trophoblastic thesis of cancer. In a review of 17,000 papers on malignant neoplasms and related biological subjects, the trophoblast was described as the *sine qua non* of cancer.[187]

RATIONALE
The malignant lesion is characterized by a high focal concentration of beta glucuronidase, which is a beta-glucosidase. Laetrile is a glucoside which is hydrolyzed specifically by beta-glucosidase enzymes, with production of benzaldehyde, glucose, and nascent hydrogen cyanide.

Rhodanese, the cyanide-detoxifying enzyme, is absent or relatively deficient in malignant lesions but present in normal tissues. Nascent hydrocyanic acid is released to the extent of about 10% in the vulnerable carcinomatous areas but not elsewhere in the body.

PREVIOUS REPORTS
In a group of 14 cases of cancer with metastases treated with Laetrile, there was striking relief of pain with discontinuance of analgesics, disappearance of fetor from ulceration, improved appetite and regression of the tumor.[188]

In another study of 21 terminal cases, the use of Laetrile provided satisfactory relief of pain, reduction of hemorrhage and jaundice,

---

[187] Krebs, E. T., Jr., Krebs, E.T., Sr., and Beard, H. H., The Unitarian or Trophoblastic Thesis of Cancer, *M. Rec.* 163: 1 5 8- 73, July, 1950

[188] Navarro, M. D., The mechanism of action and therapeutic effects of Laetrile in Cancer, *J.Philippine M. A.* 33:620-7, Aug. 1957

almost constant improvement in strength and the hematological pattern, and in sonic cases an appreciable reduction of the neoplastic mass.[189]

CLINICAL MATERIAL

The present group included 5 males and 5 females. The average age was 45, range 17 to 74. The diagnosis was adenocarcinoma of the breast 4 cases, Hodgkin's disease 3, cancer of the lung 1, cancer of the prostate 1, and cancer of the pancreas and omentum 1. Metastases were present in all cases.

Pain was a prominent symptom in all 10 cases and 7 patients required narcotics for relief.

Adenopathy was present in all cases and fetor in 1.

The average period of treatment with Laetrile was 17.5 weeks, range 4 to 43; average number of slow intravenous injections 30.2, range 6 to 79; average total dosage 46.2 Gm., range 9 to 133.

RESULTS OF TREATMENT

Dramatic relief of pain resulted in all 10 cases after the first or second slow intravenous injection and continued throughout the course of treatment. In 5 cases pain disappeared completely and in the other 5 it was definitely reduced. Narcotics were discontinued in 5 of the 7 cases in which they were used.

After 7 injections the fetor from an ulcerating adenocarcinoma of the breast disappeared and the discharge ceased.

Adenopathy was considerably reduced in 8 of the 10 cases in which it was present.

---

[189] Tasca, N., Clinical observation on the therapeutic effects of a cyanogenetic glycuronoside in cases of human malignant neoplasms, *Gazz. Med. ital.* 118:153-9, Apr. 1959

HEMOGRAM AND URINALYSIS

In all-cases except #4 and #8, the blood picture was greatly improved after use of Laetrile. There was no indication of agranulocytosis or other hematogenous toxicity.

The average red blood cell count before treatment was 3,941,000, after treatment 4,515,000 (15% increase). The average white blood cell count before treatment was 10,200, after treatment 9,750 (2% decrease, statistically insignificant). The average hemoglobin before treatment was 11.65 Gm. per 100 cc., after treatment 12.4 (6% increase). The before and after differential blood counts showed no significant changes and no abnormal blood cells were found.

Urinalysis was negative. Kidney function was not altered or affected by the use of Laetrile.

UNTOWARD REACTIONS

A sudden fall of blood pressure occurring five minutes after the injection was a common occurrence. In 1 case the drop amounted to 68 mm. and was accompanied by shock, requiring an injection of phenylephrine hydrochloride.

To avoid shock, I now use phenylephrine hydrochloride 0.3 mg. routinely in the same syringe with the Laetrile solution. This precaution has proved effective in maintaining a stable blood pressure during and after injections of Laetrile.

DISCUSSION

Laetrile is not a general analgesic *per se*, although on hydrolysis it releases a small amount of benzoic acid which is analgesic. Therefore the consistent relief of pain and discontinuance of narcotics after one or two injections, lasting throughout the course of treatment, are significant results. The sudden disappearance of fetor and discharge from ulcerating adenocarcinoma of the breast and reduction of adenopathy are also encouraging.

It would appear that Laetrile injections cause a regression of the malignant lesion. More cases and a follow-up study are required to evaluate the degree and permanence of this result. The findings present an image of cancer which is consistent with the trophoblastic thesis.

CASE REPORTS

Case 1. W.L., age 62, female, married, housewife, weight 118 lb., height 62 in., blood pressure 144/95 mm. Diagnosis: adenocarcinoma of both breasts with metastases to the skull, pelvis and spine. There was bilateral inguinal adenopathy. History of bilateral mastectomy, eighteen years apart, followed by deep X-ray therapy. Urinalysis and hematology negative.

During the last six months the patient had suffered from constant excruciating pain in the back, entire spinal region, pelvis, thighs and legs. She was unable to lie down and tried to sleep in a chair. Repeated doses of codeine and other analgesics every two or three hours were required.

Laetrile 1 Gm. was injected intravenously. In five minutes the systolic blood pressure dropped 12 mm. but there were no other apparent effects. The following day the patient walked into my office without aid and reported that she had slept well with very little pain, that she needed less codeine, and that her appetite was good. Her general appearance was greatly improved.

An injection of Laetrile 1 Gm. was repeated. The systolic blood pressure fell 10 mm, but there were no apparent side-effects. After ten minutes she said that pain was relieved completely and stepped down from the examining table without help.

In a period of one month she received six injections of Laetrile, four of 1 Gm. and two of 2 Gm. In each instance there was a prompt fall of blood pressure, average 10.4 mm., range 8-12 mm.

During the period of treatment the patient returned to her housework, was almost free from pain, discontinued codeine, took no analgesics other than 10 grains of aspirin at bedtime or during the night, and slept well. Her morale was excellent, her appetite good, and she gained 31/2 lb. At the last examination she reported that she was completely free from pain. There were no apparent adverse effects from any of the injections. As of May 1, 1962 the hemogram showed distinct improvement in red blood cell count and hemoglobin, with no adverse change. Urinalysis was negative.

Case 2. J.S., age 74, male, married, pattern maker, weight 163 lb, height 62 in., blood pressure 188/100 mm. Diagnosis: inoperable carcinoma of the left lung with metastasis to the mediastinum. Urinalysis and hematology negative.

During the last six months the patient complained of cough, constant chest pain, dyspnea, blood-tinged expectoration, anorexia, and loss of weight (15 lbs.). An X-ray revealed a mass in the left side of the chest suggestive of a neoplasm. Bronchoscopy and a biopsy established the diagnosis of carcinoma of the lung. Exploratory thoracotomy showed extensive carcinoma of the left lung with metastases and many perforations in the pleura, diaphragm, aorta, pericardium and mediastinum. The condition was considered inoperable.

Pain was so constant and severe that the patient took meperidine hydrochloride and codeine every two or three hours. When interviewed, he had such great difficulty in talking and breathing that his wife had to give the history.

Physical examination revealed icteric sclerae, pallid conjunctivae, sluggish reflexes, enlarged and tender cervical and supraclavicular glands, dullness and moist rales over the left of the chest, and edema of the ankles extending up to the knees.

Laetrile 1 Gm. was injected intravenously. In five minutes the systolic blood pressure dropped 28 mm., but there were no signs of shock or other adverse effects. Three days later the patient reported that the pain had been less severe since the injection, but that he had suffered for two days from pain in the left shoulder and side of the chest. Analgesics were still required.

After the second intravenous injection of Laetrile 1 Gm., the systolic blood pressure fell 15 mm. but there were no side-effects other than burning and itching in the left shoulder area. One week later the patient returned to the office unassisted. Pain, dyspnea and edema were considerably diminished. His color and general appearance were considerably improved.

In a period of seven weeks he received sixteen injections of Laetrile, seven of 1 Gm., six of 1.5 Gm., and three of 2 Gm. There was a prompt fall of blood pressure following the injections, ranging from 8 to 28 mm. Pain was reduced and appetite improved but there was no weight gain. He was able to discontinue use of meperidine hydrochloride and codeine. There were no apparent adverse effects from the injections as shown by the before and after hemograms and urinalyses.

Case 3. J.C., age 40, female, married, house-wife, weight 113 lb., height 61 in, blood pressure 140/90 mm. Diagnosis: infiltrating carcinoma of the left breast invading the lymphnodes at all levels of the axilla, with metastases to the liver. Radical mastectomy and deep X-ray therapy. Urinalysis and hematology negative.

For the last six months she had suffered from very severe pain in the abdomen and back. Meperidine hydrochloride, morphine and opium were required for relief.

Laetrile 1 Gm. was injected intravenously. In five minutes the systolic blood pressure dropped 10 mm. but there were no other apparent effects. She returned the following day and reported no relief of pain.

An intravenous injection of Laetrile 1 Gm. was repeated, following when the systolic blood pressure dropped 12 mm. There was considerable reduction of pain and appetite improved after this injection.

In a period of four weeks she received twelve injections of Laetrile, ten of 1 Gm. and two of 1.5 Gm. Pain was relieved almost entirely and only a single dose of narcotic drug at bedtime was required. Morale and appetite were improved but there was no gain in weight. There were no apparent adverse effects from the injections. Comparison of before and after hemograms showed improvement in the red blood cell count and hemoglobin following Laetrile therapy.

Case 4. J.F., age 38, female, married house-wife, weight 155 lb., height 62 in., blood pressure 160/90 mm. Diagnosis: adenocarcinoma of left breast with carcinomatosis. Mastectomy, deep X-ray therapy and castration. Urinalysis and hematology negative.

The patient complained of agonizing pain in her spine, chest, pelvis, legs, arms and head. X-ray visualization confirmed the diagnosis of disseminated metastases. Adenopathy was present. Codeine, meperidine hydrochloride and opium were required to control the pain.

Laetrile 1 Gm. was injected intravenously. After fifteen minutes the systolic blood pressure rose 3 mm. There were no apparent side-effects. On the following day pain was reduced, appetite improved, and the general condition was somewhat better.

A second intravenous injection of Laetrile 1 Gm. was given. In five minutes the systolic blood pressure dropped 16 mm. but there were no apparent side-effects. Three days later the patient reported that the pain was considerably less and she required a minimum dosage of opiates for relief.

In a period of eighteen days she received eight injections of Laetrile, five of 1 Gm., two of 1.5 Gm and 1 of 2 Gm. During the period of medication she showed progressive improvement and suffered very little pain. Opiates were no longer required. Morale was excellent. There were no apparent adverse effects from the injections. Comparison of before and after hemograms showed improvement in the red blood cell count and hemoglobin following Laetrile therapy.

Case 5. R.F., age 20, male, single, premedical student, weight 200 lb., height 59 in., blood pressure 114/70 mm. Diagnosis: malignant lymphoma, type Hodgkin's. Condition started as enlarged cervical gland, diagnosis on biopsy. Urinalysis negative, hemoglobin 11 Gm./100cc.

Deep X-ray therapy was employed. The patient complained of weakness, dizziness, and pain in the axillae and groin. The cervical, axillary and inguinal glands were palpably enlarged. The conjunctivae and sclerae were pale and icteric.

Laetrile 1 Gm. was injected intravenously. In ten minutes the systolic blood pressure dropped 6 mm. but there were no other apparent effects. Four days later the patient reported that he felt more active, had a better appetite, and had suffered no ill-effects.

An injection of Laetrile 1Gm. was repeated. The systolic blood pressure dropped 4 mm. in ten minutes, no other apparent effects.

In a period of four and a half months he received nineteen injections of Laetrile, five of 1 Gm. and fourteen of 2 Gm.

During the period of medication the pains in the neck and groin ceased and the adenopathy disappeared. The patient felt euphoric and his general appearance was considerably improved. There were no apparent adverse effects from the injections. The blood picture improved after Laetrile therapy.

Case 6. L.D., age 47, female, single, draftsman, weight 190 lb., height 66 in., blood pressure 280/110 mm. Diagnosis infiltrating adenocarcinoma of left breast. Both her mother and sister had died of cancer. History of radical mastectomy. Metastases in left axilla broke down, producing multiple sinuses.

The principal complaints were severe pain in the left side of the chest, necessitating the use of codeine, and a foul odor from the discharging sinuses. To control her distressing cough it was necessary to prescribe meperidine hydrochloride and opium for use on alternate days.

The left shoulder and arm were swollen and painful. The skin was glistening red. The circumference of the left mid-arm measured 19 ¾ ins. as compared with 13 ins. for the right. Adenopathy was present in the entire left axillary and supraclavicular areas, both sides of the neck, and in the right breast. The liver was palpable and tender. Both sides of the chest were tender and especially painful on coughing.

Laetrile 1 Gm. was injected intravenously. In five minutes the systolic blood pressure dropped 38 mm. but there were no apparent other effects. On the following day she received a second injection. Pain and cough diminished and there was less discharge from the axillary sinuses. However, she felt a sense of heat and itching in the operative area. After the third injection pain was relieved completely and the fetor disappeared. After the fourth injection, the drainage ceased completely and the area was odorless. Multiple crusts covered the healing sinuses. Induration and inflammation were almost completely gone. The texture of the skin of the left arm had returned to normal.

In a period of five months she received fifty injections of Laetrile, nine of 1 Gm., thirty-nine of 2 Gm., and two of 2.5 Gm. The immediate hypotensive response was easily controlled when phenylephrine hydrochloride 0.3 mg. Was used simultaneously with Laetrile.

During the period of treatment the patient returned to work. Pain and cough disappeared. The discharge from the metastatic sinuses ceased and there was no more fetor. The circumference of the left mid-arm was reduced from 19 3/4 in. to 17 in., an indication of less tumefaction. Narcotics for relief of pain and cough were no longer required. There were no apparent adverse effects from any of the injections.

In this case treatment with Laetrile was continued from July 7, 1961 until May 1962. In the extended period of ten months the patient received 133 injections, twice a week or more often. Comparison of before and after hemograms showed definite improvement in the red blood cell counts and hemoglobin. Adenopathy and tumefaction regressed to a considerable extent.

Case 7. G.P., age 21, male, single, college student, weight 149 lb., height 70 in., blood pressure 110/70 mm. Diagnosis: malignant lymphoma, Hodgkins type. Urinalysis and hematology negative.

A growing mass in front of the right ear, which returned four years after its initial appearance and recession, was removed and found to contain multinucleated giant cells typical of Hodgkin's disease. There was a hard, tender, enlarged lymph node in the mid-sternocleidomastoid region measuring 3x2cm. Urinalysis and liematology were negative.

Laetrile 1 Gm. was injected intravenously. The systolic blood pressure dropped 4 mm. but there were no apparent side-effects. Three days later the enlarged gland was smaller, softer, and less painful. By the sixth day all pain had ceased.

In a period of four months he received twenty-seven injections of Laetrile, ten of 1Gm. and seventeen of 2 Gm. There were no side-effects. One injection, made directly into the tumor mass, was followed by itching and local tenderness.

During the period of treatment the patient returned to college. Pain was absent, appetite good, weight increased 13 lb., and his appearance was excellent. The blood picture improved under Laetrile therapy.

Case 8. A.T., age 66, male, married, fireman, weight 120 lb., height 68 in., blood pressure 188/98 mm.. Diagnosis inoperable carcinoma of the prostate with possible metastasis to the liver. hemoglobin 10 Gm./100 cc.

The patient complained of nocturia hematuria, nausea vomiting, and severe pain in the groin and thighs. Codeine and meperidine hydrochloride were required for relief. The skin and sclerac were jaundiced. There was painful adenopathy in both groins.

Laetrile 1 Gm. was injected intravenously. In seven minutes the blood pressure dropped 68 mm. and the skin became cold and clammy. The patient appeared to be in incipient shock but responded promptly to an injection of phenylephrine hydrochloride, after which his blood pressure recovered 66 mm.

Next day an injection of Laetrile 1 Gm. was repeated. His systolic blood pressure dropped 10 mm. but there was no shock reaction.

Following the second injection the pain ceased and the use of narcotics was no longer needed. Nausea and vomiting were relieved, and jaundice was reduced.

In a period of four days he received three injections of Laetrile 1 Gm. During this time there was no pain and narcotic drugs were discontinued. Bleeding from the bladder ceased. Nausea and vomiting were relieved, and jaundice was diminished. Before and after hemograms and urinalyses showed no change.

Case 9. M.T., age 65, female, married, housewife, weight 110 lb., height 66 in., blood pressure 160/90 mm. Diagnosis: adenocarcinoma of the pancreas and omentum. Hemoglobin 11.5 Gm./100cc. The liver was palpable and painful nodules extended to about 3 inches below the costal margin.

During the last seven months she had suffered from extreme pain and had lost 20 lb. Meperidine hydrochloride was required for relief. She was exceedingly weak, jaundiced, emaciated, and unable to stand without assistance.

Laetrile 1 Gm. was injected intravenously. There were no adverse effects. A second injection was given four days later.

Pain was partially relieved and the dosage of meperidine hydrochloride was reduced. The blood picture and urinalysis showed no change under Laetrile therapy.

Case 10. F.F- Age 17, male, single, student. weight 140 lb., height 71 in., blood pressure 110/70. Diagnosis: Hodgkin's disease, granuloma type, with metastasis to the thorax.

During the last three months a growing mass in the left supraclavicular region had reached the size of a quarter sphere of an average orange. The patient complained of pain in both axillae, weakness, nausea and anorexia. He had lost 25lb. and was jaundiced. Biopsy confirmed the diagnosis. The axillary lymph glands were enlarged, especially on the right side. The roentgenograms showed progressive nodal enlargement inside the thorax.

Laetrile 1 Gm. was injected intravenously. In five minutes the systolic blood pressure dropped 6 mm. but there were no apparent other effects.

On examination two days later the mass in the neck was softer and smaller. By the fifth day it was reduced to about half the original size, and was softer and movable. The axillary lymph glands were barely palpable. He was free from pain and his appetite had returned.

In a period of five months he received thirty-six injections of Laetrile, nineteen of 1 Gm. and seventeen of 2 Gm. There were no side-effects.

During the period of treatment there was no pain and no enlargement of the supraclavicular mass occurred. Appetite improved and the patient gained 24 lb. He returned to his studies. Comparison of before and after hemograms showed distinct improvement in the red blood cell count and hemoglobin.

SUMMARY
The use of Laetrile (1-mandelonitrile-beta-glycuronoside), a beta cyanogenetic glucoside, intravenously in 10 cases of inoperable cancer, all with metastases, provided dramatic relief of pain, discontinuance of narcotics, control of fetor, improved appetite, and reduction of adenopathy. The results suggest regression of the malignant lesion.

A fall of blood pressure occurred in all cases after administration of Laetrile. This side-effect was easily avoided by using phenylephrine hydrochloride 0.3-1 mg. in the same syringe with the Laetrile solution. No other side-effects were noted except slight itching and a sensation of heat in the affected areas, which was transitory in all cases.

Comparison of before and after hemograms showed definite improvement in the red blood cell count and hemoglobin in most cases. Differential blood counts and urinalyses were entirely negative.

PRELIMINARY OBSERVATIONS OF CANCER CASES TREATED WITH LAETRILE

Ettore Guidetti
Professor of Pharmacology
University of Turin Medical School

Presented at the Sixth International Cancer Congress
Sao Paulo, Brazil, July 1954

Translated from the French by Credence Research

Krebs and his colleagues have recently considered the possibility that cyanogenetic glycuronsides could have a certain palliative effect on human cancers. The theoretical foundation of this assertion is based on the following findings:

a) Neoplastic tissues are characterized by a very clear beta-glycuronidase activity, which appears to be in direct link to their degree of malignancy. (Fishman; Fishman and Anlyan; Odell, Bury and Bethea; Anlyan, Gamble and Hoster; Campbell; Seligmann, Nachlas, Manheimer, Friedman and Wolf; Homburger and Fishman);[190]

b) On the other hand neoplastic tissues are characterized by very weak activity of the enzyme rhodanese (transsulferase), which can transform hydrocyanic acid into rhodanates. (Lang; Summer and Somers; Mendel, Rodney and Bowman; Gal, Fung and Grunberg);[191]

c) Cyanogenetic glycuronosides are able to emit HCN due to the effect of beta-glycuronidases on beta-glucosidases, either in vitro or in vivo. (Krebs et al; McIlroy);[192]

d) Normal tissues which contain beta-glycuronidases, also contain sufficient quantities of rhodaneses, as opposed to neoplastic tissues, and are able to detoxify the HCN emitted

---

[190] Krebs Jr., Krebs Sr., Bartlett, Bodman, Harris, Malin and Beard, 1 (1954); Fishman: *Science*, 105, 646, 1947; Fishman and Anlyan: *Science*, 106, 66,1947. *J. Biol. Chem.*, 1969, 449, 1947. Forth Int. Cancer Research Cong. 6,1034,1950; Odell, Burt and Berthea: *Cancer Research,* 9,362,1949; Anylan, Gamble and Horter: *Cancer*, 3,116, 1950; Campbell: *Brit. J. Exper. Path.*, 30,548, (1949); Seligmann, Nachlas, Manheimer, Friedman and Wolf: *Ann. Surg.*, 130,133,1939; Homburger and Fishman: "The Physiopathology of Cancer", P. Hoeber, N.Y., 91953

[191] Lang: *Bioch.* Z.259. 243,1933; Summer and Somers: Chemistry and Methods of Enzymes. Academic Press, N.Y. (1947); Mendel, Rodney and Bowman: *Cancer Research*, 6,495,1946; Gal, Fung and Greenberg: *Cancer Research,* 12,565,1952

[192] Krebs Jr., Krebs Sr., Bartlett, Bodman, Harris, Malin and Beard, 1 (1954); Fishman: *Science*, 105, 646, 1947; McIlroy: The plant glucosides. E. Arnold, London, (1952)

by the hydrolysis of cyanogenetic beta-glycuronosides by transforming it into rhodanates. (Bernard, Gajdos and Gaddos-Torok; Sanchez, Bertran and Vilas);[193]

e) The neoplastic cells appear to have a selective sensitivity to HCN. (Karczag and Gsab; Maxwell and Bishoff; Perry).[194]

In the light of these findings Krebs et al propose a medical treatment of cancer with the help of cyanogenetic glycuronsides, given that an excess of free HCN could be emitted at the level of neoplastic tissues due to the effect of beta-glycuronidases on glycuronosides, which cannot be detoxified by the absence of rhodanese, and given the particular sensitivity of neoplastic cells to HCN.

Cyanogenetic glycuronside developed for therapeutic use is the l-mandelo-nitrile beta-glucuronside, and is either prepared synthetically or bio-synthetically from amygdalin: through enzymatic hydrolysis, it can emit HCN, glycuronic acid and benzaldehyde which is immediately oxidised into benzoic acid; the cyanhydric acid can be detoxified into rhodanate by the rhodanese in normal tissues, while it could develop its toxic effect on neoplastic tissues, which are lacking in rhodanese.

According to this notion, the cyanogenetic glycuronoside can be viewed as strictly chemotherapeutic medicine, elective vis à vis neoplastic cells, since it is able to emit, on the level of these pathological tissues, a very toxic element such as HCN, which cannot be detoxified by enzymatic means and for this reason it can play its destructive role in the neoplastic cells: that is to say an eminently tropic-cancer effect, and almost not tropic-organo, according to Erhlich's classic theory.

Although therapeutics of the administration of cyanogenetic glycuronoside have been proposed by parenteral means (intra-

---

[193] Genard, Gajdos and Gajdos-Torok: *Rev. Path. Comparee*, 49,72,1949; Sanchez, Bertran and Vilas: *Anal, Fac.Vetuniv.* Madrid, 2,97,1950
[194] Karczag and Csaba, *Med.Klin*, 23,1413,1927; Maxwell and Bishoff: *J. Pharm. Exp.Ther.*, 49,240,1933; Perry, *Am.J. Cancer*,25,592,1935

muscular injection), in the aim of directly controlling the lytic and destructive effect vis à vis the neoplastic tissues of these substances, I have applied a topical treatment, with dressings in situ, for external ulcerated neoplasms, or those directly accessible from the surface.

I have subjected the cases of the following cancers to topical treatment with cyanogenetic glycuronoside by the name of Laetrile, a white crystalline powder, very easily dissolved in water or physiological solution: 1) cancers of the upper part of the rectum; 2) cancers of the neck of the womb; 3) ulcerated breast cancers.

The topical treatment was continued with the help of a local dressing by means of a gauze compress soaked with 20 ml of Laetrile solution (100mg up to 250mg of glycuronoside each time); the dressing stayed in situ for 24 hours and it was changed every three days. The quantity of Laetrile and the number of dressings were variable, depending on the local and general reaction of the patient.

When dealing with neoplasms of the neck of the womb or the rectum a swab saturated with Laetrile solution was introduced into the vaginal cavity or the rectum, directly in contact with the cancer, in the case of large and growing neoplasms which were easily accessible from the exterior. During the period of time when this aforesaid local treatment was being followed, all other therapeutics were suspended.

With regard to the determined effects of the topical dressings of Laetrile on neoplastic masses - effects which one could objectively control with direct vision, given the seat of the treated tumour - one could say the lytic and destructive effect of glycuronoside vis à vis the cancerous tissues has been very clear, and in certain cases one was able to observe a melting away of the neoplastic, growing mass.

With regard to the patient's reaction to the treatment, one has not only to realise that the medication could easily be absorbed through the tissues with which it has direct contact, but also that the products of the cellular disintegration, caused by the glycuronoside, will be reabsorbed. The first fact should not be determined by the general reactions of the body, since the toxic element HCN, which is given off by the medication, should be rapidly detoxified by the enzymatic effect of the rhodanese, according to theoretical assurances; while the second fact could play a determining role with regard to the general reaction to the treatment, in particular the pyretic and toxic reaction which could follow the re-absorption of waste from the cellular disintegration.

In effect, an increase in body temperature was sometimes experienced in some patients, and more rarely a transitory pyrexia accompanied by shivers and a profuse sweating in direct relation with the Laetrile dressing, which is manifested more precisely in patients where the destruction of neoplastic tissue was clearer. Apart from this pyretic reaction, treatment by topical dressing has not caused any particular secondary effects, except a burning sensation and a local discomfort.

Consequently the lytic effects determined by the Laetrile on the neoplastic tissues seem to confirm the chemotherapeutic effect of the glycuronoside, in the tropic-cancer sense.

In other respects, the cyanogenetic glycuronoside could play the same role by parenteral means, which I have had the opportunity to observe with patients carrying pulmonary neoplasms or even pulmonary metastasis. Subjected to Laetrile treatment (2g in total, by an intra-muscular injection of 100mg every four days) one has been able to note, by controlled radiography, a regression of the neoplasm or the metastasis.

CONCLUSIONS

One can recognise that topical treatment with cyanogenetic glycuronoside, otherwise known as Laetrile, of certain directly accessible human cancers produces lytic and destructive effects on neoplastic tissues, due to a mechanism of enzyme action, and as a result, one can consider the usefulness of this medical treatment for human cancers of the rectum, the neck of the womb and ulcerated cancers of the breast.

CLINICAL TRIAL OF CHEMOTHERAPEUTIC TREATMENT OF ADVANCED CANCERS WITH LAETRILE (L-MANDELONITRILE-BETA-DIGLUCOSIDE)

Benedetto Rossi
Ettore Guidetti
And
Christian Deckers

Presented at the 9th International Cancer Congress in Tokyo, October 1966

Among numerous chemotherapeutic substances suggested for the treatment of malignant neoplasm formations, we have, for approximately ten years, resorted to l-mandelonitrile-beta-glucoside (trade name LAETRILE) for a certain number of cancer carriers in the terminal stage of the disease.

Our use of this glucoside came about principally because of its low toxicity, as demonstrated by biological tests on animals: as a matter of fact the median lethal dose was 11,600 mg/KG intra-muscularly, and 9,400mg/Kg intravenously in mice - that is, approximately 800 times higher than the daily dose used in therapy, which averaged 1,000 mg per patient.

The active principle of this substance is probably its decomposition by beta-glucosidase in the cancerous tissues, with release of hydrocyanic acid in the nascent state acting toxically on the cancerous cells. This enzyme has been shown to be present in considerable quantity, especially at the level of the neoplastic tissues of the cervix uteri. (Fishman & Anylan)

We used the product in cycles of intramuscular or intravenous injections and even, in certain cases by introduction into the cervical, uterine, pleural or peritoneal cavities when neoplastic effusion occurred.

Until 1960 we administered in doses of 100mg to 500 mg dissolved in 5 ml distilled water or in 5% glucose solution; from 1960 we went on to heavier dosages, usually 1,00 mg/day, very rarely higher than that except in the case of intracavitary introduction, where doses ranged as high as 3,000 mg or 4,000 mg.

The product is generally well tolerated. However, we must point out certain cases where a side-effect at hepatocyte level was observed, enhanced by a hepatic insufficiency, syndrome and more rarely by the appearance of a form of jaundice; at the level of the kidney, at the level of the bone marrow; accompanied sometimes by deposition of a number of white corpuscles, though this was never very considerable. All these side-effects could, on the one hand, be related to the action of the product at these various tissue levels, or, on the other hand due, to the generally defective systemic status of carriers with long-term tumors, with the possible presence of hepatic metastases.

The total glucoside dosage varied from 10 to 30 grams for each course of therapy, depending on the patient's reaction or according to the side-effects or therapeutic results observed. Often several successive courses were made with the same patient.

During this therapy, symptomatic remedies (analgesics, cardiotonics, diuretics) only were administered, without recourse to any other type of chemotherapeutic or physical therapy. In the majority of patients however, we associated a kind of immunotherapy based on parenteral administration of certain extractive lipids from human neoplastic tissues, suggested by one of ourselves and dealt with in GUIDETTI and MAISIN's communication to this Congress.

In all possible cases the evolution of the disease and the therapeutic response were followed by biopsies, radiographic and haematological controls, control of sedimentation rate, and all other checks deemed necessary in each particular case. Among these latter was a test depending on deviation of complement, which allows an assessment of the immunitary response in respect of the neoplastic disease. This test, where the RNA of the aphthous fever virus is used as antigen, suggested by our Italo-Belgian working party in 1965, is discussed in a communication to this Congress by GUANINI, SERRA, GUIDETTI, MAISIN, and DECKERS, and was published in a 1966 issue of *Nature*.

From 1954 to 1966 we gave 150 patients the above-mentioned therapy, chiefly at San Cottolengo Hospital, Turin; Dosio Hospital, Milan; and Louvain University Ca· ·r Institute. All patients were in the terminal stage of the disease, the majority of them prey to cachezia, and all other therapies had failed.

The following table summarizes the cases treated, classified according to the site of the tumor, and showing the number of patients for each degree of reaction to therapy. We use the sign ++

to denote patients who reacted in an objectively favorable manner, by which we mean diminution of volume of the tumor or at least all interruption of its evolution, improvement in the roentgenographic picture, and improvement in laboratory findings. The mark + and ± indicates patients who showed a more or less distinct subjective improvement, and the mark - those who reacted negatively to the treatment.

Cases corresponding to ++ represent about 20% of those treated.

We again underline the fact that the majority of these cases were simultaneously subjected to an immunotype therapy, which might have some bearing on the number of positive results observed, grouped under the signs+ + and + totalling about half the number of cases treated.

Cancer Site	No. Cases	++	+	±	-
Toruli tactiles	26	5	6	6	9
Breast	25	3	8	7	7
Uterus	24	7	7	4	6
Rectum	20	2	9	2	7
Ovary (with infusion)	10	2	2	2	4
Other types	30	9	7	2	12
Totals	135	28	39	23	45

We have separately considered neoplasms of the pleura with effusion (15 cases), where the product was used direct by injection in the pleural cavity. In these cases we observed our best results, as generally we obtained reduction and then on occasion complete disappearance of the effusion, associated with a distinct improvement in the patients' condition.

CONCLUSION
On the basis of our clinical trial, we are able to state that l-mandelonitrile-beta-diglucoside may be considered an extremely useful chemotherapeutic drug for palliative medical treatment of

malign neoplasms, from the standpoint both of its therapeutic effect and its very low toxicity.

One of us tested the product on the cancerous cell (Ehrlich's ascites), taking as standard the inhibition of breathing measured by Warburg's method. We were able to confirm production of HCN and benzaldehyde, both toxic on the cancer cell. Presence of beta-glucosidase is essential for break-up of the product.

LAETRILE (NITRILOSIDE) BIBLIOGRAPHY

GUIDETTI, ETTORE
Observations Preliminaires Sur Quelques Cas de Cancer Traites Par Un Glycuronoside Cyanogenetique. *Acta Unio Internationalis Contra Cancrum,* XI (No. 2): 156-158 (1955). Read at the Sixth International Cancer Congress, Sao Paulo, July, 1954. (pp) *Edizioni Minerva Medica (1958). Med.,* 9; 468-471 (1954)

TASCA, MARCO
Osservazioni Cliniche Sugli Effetti Terapeutici ci un Glicuronoside cianogenetico in Casi di Neoplasie Maligne Umane. *Gazzetta Medica Italiana* (19 pp.) *Edizioni Minerva Medica.* (1958)

NAVARRO, MANUEL D.
- Laetrile – The Ideal Anti-Cancer Drug? *Santo Tomas J. Med.,* 9:468-471 (1954)
- Laetrile in Malignancy. Santo Tomas J. Med., 10:113-118 (1955).
- D. STA. ANA, J. ZANTUA and G. MORAL, Metastatic Pulmonary Carcinoma Treated with Laetrile (Report of a Case*), Unitas,* 28:606-618 (1955)
- and C. L. LAGMAN, Breast Carcinoma with Lung and Bone Metastases Treated with Laetrile (Case Report), *Santo Tomas J. Med.,* 11: 196-203 (1956); *J. Philippine Med. Assn.,*33:16-29 (1957)
- Biochemistry of Laetrile Therapy in Cancer*, Papyrus* 1:8-9, 27-28 (1957)
- Mechanism of Action and Therapeutic Effects of Laetrile in Cancer. *J. Philippine Med. Assn.,* 33:620-627 (1957)

G. GAMEZ, A. DIZON, A. PEREZ, L. MARANAN, and S. ALVAREZ
- Chemotherapy of Cancer, Laetrile in Cancers of the Throat, *Philippine J. of Cancer 1:* 131-137 (1957)

- Five Years Experience with Laetrile Therapy in Advanced Cancer, *Acta Unio internationalis Contra Cancrum, XV* (*b*is):209-221 (1959). Read at the Symposium on Cancer Chemotherapy for Pacific Asian Area, International Union Against Cancer, Tokyo, October 1957.
- Report on Proceedings of International Symposium on Cancer Chemotherapy at Tokyo, October 1957, *Santo Tomas J. med.*, 12:244-453 (1957)

F. G.GUERRERO and R. SIN
- Laetrile Therapy of Breast Cancer. *Santo Tomas J. Med.*, 13:29-36 (1958)
- Biochemical Diagnosis and Treatment of Cancer, *Unitas*, 31 (No. 2) 76 pp. (1958). Republished as a book, Manila, Univ. of Santo Tomas Press, 1958

NAVARRO, R.P.
- The Use of the Beard Anthrone Test in Certain Cases Inaccessible to or with Doubtful or Negative Biopsy. *Philippine J. of Cancer,* 2:123-136 (1958)
- Early Cancer Diagnosis with the Beard Anthrone Test (Navarro's Modification), *Philippine J. of Cancer,* 2:285-304 *1958); Acta Unio Internationalis Contra Cancrum, XVI:* 1482-1491 (1960). Read at the Seventh International Cancer Congress, London, July 1958
- The Unitarian or Trophoblastic Thesis of Cancer, *Philippine J. of Cancer* 3:3-11 (1959)
- Early Cancer Detection - A Biochemical Approach, *Santo Tomas J. Med.*, 15:111-129 (1960)
- The Role of the Chemotherapeutic Agents in Cancer. *Bulletin of the Quezon Institute*, 1960. Read at Seminar of the Quezon Institute, *Santo Tomas J. Med., 15:* 443-450 (1960)
- Early Cancer Detection. *J. Philippine Med. Assn.*, 36:425-432 (1960)
- Laetrile Therapy in Cancer. Read at the Eighth International Cancer Congress, Moscow, U.S.S.R. July 1962, *The Philippine Journal of Cancer*, July-Sept., 1962

MORRONE, JOHN A.
- Chemotherapy of Inoperable Cancer. Preliminary Report of Ten Cases Treated with Laetrile (nitriloside), *Experimental Medicine and Surgery*, #4, 1962

KREBS, ERNST T., JR., and N. R. BOUZIANE,
- Beta-Cyanophoric Glucuronosides and Glucosides (Nitrilosides). Their Rationale and Clinical Utilization in Human Cancer. *In Press.*

RESTIFO, J. A. and M. A. GAMA
- The Use of Laetrile (Nitriloside) in the Treatment of Cancer, with Case Reports. *In M.S.* (1962)

ROSSI, BENEDETTO; GUIDETTI, ETTORE and DECKERS, CHRISTIAN
- Clinical Trial of Chemotherapeutic Treatment of Advanced Cancers with l-Mandelonitrile-Beta-Diglucoside. Presented at the Ninth International Cancer Congress in Tokyo, October 1966.

HARRIS ARTHUR T.
- Possible Palliative Value of Laetrile in Human Cancer. A Preliminary Report (1953). *In M.S.*

BEASLEY, H. EARLE
- Twenty Months' Review of the Effects of Laetrile in the Palliative Treatment of Cancer (1954). Read before the American College of Osteopathic Internists Convention at Philadelphia, 1954

The foregoing references, without exception and including those from the world's most prestigious journals in the field of oncology, are positive reports on the safety and effectiveness of Laetrile (nitriloside), and describe completely non-toxic palliation and other beneficial effects of Laetrile (nitriloside) in abolishing pain and fetor where present, decreasing and eliminating the need for narcotics, and extending life-expectancy of cancer patients left terminal by surgery and/or radiation.

For the completeness of this bibliography, we also cite the single negative report on Laetrile, published ten years ago and obviously designed to disparage continued study or investigational use of Laetrile. The said single negative report on Laetrile, which is based upon the observations of unidentified investigators in unidentified institutions administering a purported "Laetrile" not obtained from the only source of the material, is to be found in *California Medicine*, 78:320 (1953).[195]

---

[195] For a fuller comment on this report and its authors, please see Day, Phillip *Cancer: Why We're Still Dying to Know the Truth*, Credence, 2000 and Griffin, G Edward *World Without Cancer*, American Press 1998

LIVING WITH THE CHEMISTRY SET
Environmental Contributions to Cancer
by Phillip Day

John Beard's work effectively states that cancer is a stem-cell healing process that has not terminated upon completion of its task. Failure to terminate in part is laid at the door of insufficient pancreatic (digestive) enzymes, responsible for demasking the pericellular coating of trophoblast cells. Experts since have laid this deficiency of enzymes primarily at the door of diets rich in animal proteins.[196]

And now we come to the environmental causes of cancer, much trivialized by the cancer establishment, which trigger healing processes in the body which do not terminate when coupled with an inadequate intake of nutrients. A brief overview of the chemical/environmental picture serves to illustrate the breadth and depth of the reform which must follow in order to eradicate cancer from the general population.

Norine Warnock lives downwind of the British Petroleum refinery and chemical plant located in Lima, Ohio:

"I have health problems and my four-year-old daughter has serious respiratory problems. Maybe those problems are not connected to BP, but maybe they are.... The guy across the street has cancer. The woman down the street has brain cancer. The woman around the corner has brain cancer. The woman who lives next door to my child's friend has cancer. The woman on the next block has breast cancer. The guy next door to her has cancer. And so does the woman next door to him. Those are just the houses I can see when I am looking out of my own front door."[197]

* * * * *

20th century civilised society manufactures and uses tens of thousands of new chemical substances every decade. From potent

---

[196] Manner, Harold W, *The Death of Cancer*, Credence, 2002
[197] *The Ecologist,* Vol. 28, ibid.

synergised pyrethrins in fly spray through petrochemical oils in soaps and gasolines across to plastics in cars and additives in foods to keep them fresher in our supermarkets for longer periods of time, societies – indeed, the new global community, as the world is now renamed – use most of these products on a daily basis. These man-made substances do not naturally exist in nature, and so, as each new product and its chemistry presents itself as a new experience for mankind's own biology, common sense would dictate that stringent tests would be in place to ensure that the substance in question can be cleared for safe usage.

Agencies, such as Britain's Environment Agency and America's Environmental Protection Agency (EPA) exist, so far as the public is concerned, for no other reason than to ensure that we can raise our families and work at our jobs in, as far as possible, a contamination-free environment. All technologically advanced nations have such environmental agencies, and yet every year, people still die by the hundreds of thousands, polluted and poisoned by these substances. So what has gone so very wrong?

The major problem stems from the rate at which new chemicals and chemical products are pouring onto the world's markets. Government agencies, already so tightly controlled financially with annual budget constraints, simply do not have the resources to test everything. Therefore they must rely heavily on industry-sponsored reports on product safety *from the manufacturers themselves*, which naturally opens up a wide arena for abuse. Agencies such as the EPA threaten dire fines on pharmaceutical and chemical companies found indulging in any foul play in order to ram potentially unsafe products through regulation. But prosecution of such cases by government on a realistic scale is rare since litigation consumes prodigious amounts of taxpayers' money.

This dangerous, if intriguing problem has provoked an angry backlash from 'green-minded' citizens and has led to the formation of other more independent watchdogs, who in turn write their own reports. America's Center for Public Integrity (CPI) recently issued a report appropriately entitled: *Toxic Deception: How the Chemical Industry Manipulates Science, Bends the Law, and Endangers Your Health*. This slamming indictment on the world's

Industrial/Chemical Complex was authored by *Newsday* reporter Dan Fagin and *National Law Journal's* Marianne Lavelle. The bottom line of the report's conclusion confirmed what was already known: that the chemical industry was largely self-regulatory. But another more sinister dimension emerged. Namely, that safety studies performed by chemical industry sponsors tended to find chemicals innocent of health risks to the public while non-chemical researchers invariably found substantial risks associated with these same substances.

In the area of pesticides, Fagin's CPI report states that 90% of America's 1650 'weed' scientists rely heavily on grants from pesticide manufacturers. Usually these men and women are the very researchers running studies on new pesticides products for the government! These industry reports are taken seriously by the US government, which has largely adopted the line that a chemical is safe unless proven otherwise.

Russell Mokhiber, editor of *Corporate Crime Reporter* (Washington DC), has made a detailed study of the CPI report. He states:

"In 1991 and 1992, when the [US government's] *Environmental Protection Agency offered amnesty from big-money fines to any manufacturer who turned in health studies that they should have provided under the law earlier, more than 10,000 studies suddenly appeared, showing that their products already on the market pose a substantial risk."*[198]

The CPI report was highly critical of the EPA's efforts to police private laboratories that conduct important safety tests. The Center for Public Integrity's executive director Charles Lewis tells us: *"The EPA has never inspected about 1,550 of the 2,000 labs doing the manufacturer-funded studies that the EPA uses to decide whether chemicals are safe. The EPA, which does not do its own safety tests, has audited only about 3.5% of the hundreds of thousands of studies that have been submitted to the agency."*

---

[198] Mokhiber, Russell "Objective" Science at Auction, *The Ecologist,* Vol. 28, No.2, March/April 1998

CPI also discovered many revolving doors between the US government and the chemical industry. Of 344 lobbyists and lawyers who admitted to working within the chemical industry and trade associations between 1990 and 1995, at least 135 originally came from federal agencies or congressional offices. More than this, a substantial number of senior EPA officials working in toxics and pesticides for the government were later found to have left government employment to take up related positions within the chemical industry. Lewis remarks: *"There are many tales of former US officials helping the industry to thwart federal government oversight."*

Russell Mokhiber again: *"At least 3,363 trips were taken between March 1993 and March 1995 by EPA officials that were paid for – to the tune of $3 million – by corporations, universities, trade associations, environmental organizations and private sponsors.... Members of Congress have also been courted by chemical companies. The manufacturers of alachor, atrazine, formaldehyde and perchloroethylene provided 214 free trips to members of Congress and flew one key committee chairman to Rio de Janeiro."*[199]

The Toxic Substances Control Act was passed by Congress in 1976. The aim of this law was to decide which of the 70,000-plus substances in public use should be tested for toxicity. Once again, it must be stressed that even the United States federal government, with its limited funding in this area, has scant resources to conduct a large number of its own safety tests. In spite of this fact, the National Toxicology Program (NTP) was set up, involving eight federal agencies, specifically to test for carcinogenic properties of selected substances. The reality of the NTP is that only a few dozen target chemicals are tested each year in any detail. Researcher Peter Montague argues that even these tests are useless, since they do not examine the effects of these substances on the nervous system, the endocrine system, the immune system and on major organs, such as the heart, liver, lungs, kidney and brain. He writes:

---

[199] Mokhiber, Russell, ibid.

"During a typical year, while the National Toxicology Program is studying the cancer effects of one or two dozen chemicals, about 1,000 new chemicals enter commercial markets. Our federal government is simply swamped by new chemicals and cannot keep up. Furthermore, it is highly unlikely that this situation will change. No one believes that our government – or anyone else – will ever have the capacity to evaluate fully the dangers of 1,000 new chemicals each year, especially not in combination with the 70,000 chemicals already in circulation."[200]

And if the EPA gets cute with any of the major chemical corporations, Montague continues, lawyers acting for the chemical industry know they can tie up the EPA in long and expensive legal snarls for decades. The idea that government can regulate big business is ridiculous, he concludes. *"We could multiply the size of our federal government by ten (a truly frightening thought), and it would still be no match for the Fortune 500."*

Most who have studied the situation in some detail have concluded that a health disaster of monumental proportions will probably be the only way to compel a strategic change in public thinking. The chemical industry will never gain an instant morality. Ross Hume Hall makes this comment:

"We find ourselves in a similar position to that of our nineteenth century forebears. The major health issue then was infectious disease. They had no cure for typhoid or cholera, but instead launched vast public health programs of clean water, uncontaminated food and better living conditions, which eliminated much of the disease then burdening 19th century society. Such programs proved that human suffering due to illness and premature death, not to mention the medical-care costs, can be reduced or eliminated by effective social policy."[201]

---

[200] Montague, Peter edits the Environmental Research Foundation's weekly publication, *Rachel's Environment and Health Weekly*, PO Box 5036, Annapolis, MD 21403-70336 USA

[201] Hall, Ross Hume, ibid.

Standing in the dawn of this new millennium, our world faces an unprecedented crisis with its environment. Diseases that were all but unknown before the Industrial Revolution are now marching in step with our rapacious delight in stretching the control-bounds of our biotechnology. Cancer, multiple sclerosis, AIDS, ME (chronic fatigue), Alzheimers, diabetes, Parkinsons, coronary heart disease are all illnesses familiar to us, striking down family and friends with such grim reality that few expect these days to die of 'natural causes'. But are we just the innocent bystanders?

We fill our tooth cavities with mercury amalgam, a slow-release neurotoxic metal.[202] We cook our food in aluminium pots and pans and spray aluminium compounds directly into our lymph-nodes. We drink sugar-laced sodas from aluminium cans in scant disregard of the connections aluminium has with Alzheimer's Disease. We allow our drinking water to be laced with chlorine and highly dangerous hexafluorosilicic acid, toxic industry waste (this substance is generically referred to as 'fluoride'). The very food we eat has become corrupted by organophosphates, permeated with pesticides, stripped of minerals and now is increasingly genetically modified.[203]

The average apple sold off the supermarket shelf we will have saturated with chlorpyrifos, captan, iprodione, vinclozolin and then sealed in wax for longer shelf life. These pesticides, when tested, have variously caused birth defects, cancer, impaired immune response, fungal growth, genetic damage and disruption to the endocrine system. The average vitamin-depleted white bread roll can be tested positive for pesticides such as chlorpyrifos-methyl, endosulfasulphate, chlorothalonil, dothiocarbamates, iprodione, procymidone and vinclozolin.[204]

---

[202] Some Mexico cancer clinics, such as the Oasis Hospital, commence a patient's Laetrile cancer therapy by first removing all mercury amalgam fillings and replacing them with non-toxic substitutes. For a fuller treatment on the dangers of current dental techniques and what can be done, see Kellner-Read, Bill *Toxic Bite*, Credence, 2001 (available through www.credence.org)

[203] Day, Phillip *Health Wars*, Credence, 2001

[204] *The New Zealand Total Diet Survey*, 1990/1

Whilst living in Southern California, I witnessed the population of the Southland being routinely sprayed with malathion from helicopters originating from a covert government base at Evergreen, Arizona. Malathion is an organophosphate which can cause gene and immune system damage, behavioural deficits in newborns and small children, is a suspect viral enhancer and implicated in Reye's Syndrome. The purpose of the spraying is to kill the Mediterranean fruit fly which, for some inexplicable reason, prefers the concrete jungle of Los Angeles, East LA and South Pasadena to its indigenous habitat among the orchards and green pastures of central California to the north. The malathion warnings would go out over the radio: *"Cover up your cars and take your pets indoors, folks. But don't worry, it won't hurt you."*

"Milk – It Does a Body Good". Who are we kidding with what is fed to the average cow today (including steroids, antibiotics, human sewage and food fillers such as sawdust, concrete dust and paper)? Beef, pork, chicken and lamb read like a *Who's Who* of mankind's latest bold advances in steroid-bolstered, hormone-accelerated quota production. If we are what we eat, then apparently man is indeed taking a quantum step in DEvolution.

The majority of illnesses striking us today are metabolic and toxin-related in origin, which our establishment attempts to combat with the drugs and chemicals it has been trained to research and dispense. But metabolic diseases, as we know, can only be successfully regressed with metabolic preventatives, or food factors, which themselves provide the establishment with scant opportunity for profit, since they cannot be proprietarily owned or patented. Worse, the very government regulatory agencies themselves, such as the US Food & Drug Administration and Britain's Medicines Control Agency (MCA), which are supposed to protect the public from potentially dangerous products coming onto the market, are horribly compromised because of personal investments or ties with the chemical/drug industries. A USA TODAY analysis of financial conflicts at 159 FDA advisory committee meetings from 1st January to 30th June 2000 finds that:

- At 92% of the meetings, at least one member had a financial conflict of interest.

- At 55% of meetings, half or more of the FDA advisers had conflicts of interest.
- Conflicts were most frequent at the 57 meetings when broader issues were discussed: 92% of members had conflicts.
- At the 102 meetings dealing with the fate of a specific drug, 33% of the experts had a financial conflict.[205]

"The best experts for the FDA are often the best experts to consult with industry," says FDA senior associate commissioner Linda Suydam, who is in charge of waiving conflict-of-interest restrictions. But Larry Sasich of Public Citizen, an advocacy group, says, *"The industry has more influence on the process than people realize."*

Britain's Medicines Control Agency fares little better with its track record for impartiality when it comes to regulating the drug industry. According to a *Daily Express* investigation, key members of the Committee on Safety of Medicines and the Medicines Commission themselves have heavy personal investments in the drug industry. Yet these committees are the ones which decide which drugs are allowed onto the market and which are rejected!

According to the report, two thirds of the 248 experts sitting on the Medicines Commission have financial ties to the pharmaceutical industry. Drug regulators such as Dr Richard Auty have £110,000 worth of holdings with AstraZeneca. Dr Michael Denham owns £115,000 worth of shares in SmithKline Beecham. Dr Richard Logan has up to £30,000 shares in AstraZeneca, SmithKline Beecham and Glaxo Wellcome. Logan's role with the committee involves examining cases where a drug might have to be withdrawn from the market for safety reasons.

David Ganderton was an advisor for nine years with the CSM panel who used to work for AstraZeneca. His current shareholding with this drug company is worth £91,000. Other members of the committees with substantial holdings for example include Dr Colin

---

[205] *USA Today* article by Dennis Cauchon, *FDA Advisers Tied to Industry*, 25th September 2000, http://www.usatoday.com/news/washdc/ncssun06.htm

Forfar, with £22,000 with Glaxo Wellcome and Dr Brian Evans owning £28,000 worth of shares with Glaxo Wellcome.[206]

The Daily Express report goes on to tell us: *"Tom Moore, a former senior executive with AstraZeneca, told the Sunday Express that the drug companies go out of their way to build strong links. He said, "Their objective is to get as close as possible. They are an extremely powerful lobby group because they have unlimited resources."*

The [drug] *companies provide* [members of CSM and other regulatory committees] *trips abroad to conferences, large research grants that can keep a university department employed for years, and consultancies that can boost an academic's humble income."*

On the other hand, it is quite easy to understand why nutritional treatments and preventative medicine pose such a threat to this massively funded industry surrounding sickness and why they are almost never used as the primary therapy. One drug alone can cost over $200 million to go through regulation in America. Who is ever going to recoup such a cost with a vitamin or herbal treatment that cannot be patented? And herein lies the problem deadlocking Western healthcare's ability to halt Western diseases. Most of these diseases killing us are metabolic- or toxin-related and by their very definition cannot be treated with drugs or other proprietary therapies such as radiation. Yet patented treatments form the bulwark of Western medicine's tremendous wealth and power! This is the reason why Western healthcare is conspicuously failing to halt killers such as heart disease or cancer. The desire for profit is the real reason doctors receive no formal training in nutrition. The real remedies and preventatives have little or no commercial value.

Now we are in a position to see clearly why isolated tribes like the Hunzas, living in a non-industrialised environment, breathing pollution-free air, drinking chemical-free water, exercising regularly and eating wholesome fruits and vegetables rich in minerals and B17 nitrilosides, can remain free of the degenerative

---

[206] *Daily Express* micro edition, 6th August 2000

illnesses that are literally killing the 'civilised' human race around them.

THE NATURAL WAY
An Overview of Food Habits
by Phillip Day

"Most of what you have heard over your lifetime about [orthodox] *cancer treatments is not the truth. At the very least, you have received an incomplete picture. If you believe the propaganda you have been fed and you develop cancer, it can cost you your life."*
John Diamond MD

Tribes like the Abkhasians, the Azerbaijanis, the Hunzas, the Eskimaux and the Karakorum all live on nitriloside-rich food[207] and report not a single recognised case of cancer during the extended periods they have been studied by western gerontologists.

I was interviewed by radio station KFM in Tonbridge, England. The news reporter who did the interview was from the Karakorum tribe of Pakistan. She could verify that her people lived in many cases to great ages because of their diet. Their food is taken variously from buckwheat, peas, broad beans, lucerne, turnips, lettuce, sprouting pulse or gram, apricots with their seeds and berries of various kinds[208]. Their diet can be carrying as much as 250–3,000mg of nitriloside in a daily ration. The average western diet contains less than 2mg of nitriloside a day. Interestingly, natives of these tribes, who move into urban, 'civilised' areas and change their diets accordingly, always begin to fall foul of cancer at the regular western incidence. [209]

Krebs reports, concerning his studies into the dietary habits of these tribes: *"Upon investigating the diet of these people, we found that the seed of the apricot was prized as a delicacy and that every part of the apricot was utilized. We found that the major source of fats used for cooking was the apricot seed, and that the apricot oil*

---

[207] Foods rich in Vitamin B17.
[208] All these foods, with the exception of lettuce and turnips, contain high quantities of nitriloside.
[209] Stefansson, Vilhjalmur *CANCER: Disease of Civilisation? An Anthropological and Historical Study*, Hill & Wang, New York, 1960.

was so produced as inadvertently to admit a fair concentration of nitriloside or traces of cyanide into it."[210]

Western gerontologists have long studied such tribes in order to isolate the factors that appear to keep them free of degenerative diseases. Nobel laureate Dr Albert Schweitzer remarked in 1913:

"On my arrival in Gabon, I was astonished to encounter no case of cancer."[211]

Dr Stanislas Tancho, addressing the Academy of Sciences in 1843, repeated the remarks of a Doctor Bac, working as surgeon-in-chief of the Second African Regiment, who failed to come across even one case of cancer in Senegal. The surgeon-in-chief at Val-de-Grace in Algiers, a M. Baudens, was also mentioned by Dr Tancho. Baudens had worked for eight years in Algiers, coming across only two cases of cancer.[212]

James South remarks: *"Of course, such high nitriloside foods as cassava, millet, maize and sorghum are staples of the traditional African diet. Cassava may contain from 225 to 1,830 mg/kg of the nitriloside linamarin."*[213]

Concerning the Thlinget Eskimos of Alaska, the Reverend Livingston French Jones wrote in 1914:

"While certain diseases have always been found among the Thlingets, others that now afflict them are of recent introduction.

---

[210] Krebs, Ernst T *Nutritional and Therapeutic Implications*, John Beard Memorial Foundation (privately published), 1964
[211] Berglas, Alexander Preface to *Cancer: Nature, Cause and Cure,* Paris, 1957
[212] Tancho, Stanislas *Memoir on the Frequency of Cancer* (1843), quoted by Stefansson
[213] South, J, ibid; also Culbert, M, *What the Medical Establishment Won't Tell You...* ibid. Linamarin would later be used by researchers at Imperial College, London, to provide startling success in regressing cancers in tests reported in the *Daily Telegraph* and London *Times* on 6th September 2000. This news was predictably heralded as 'the latest breakthough" in cancer research.

Tumours, cancers and toothache were unknown to them until within recent years."[214]

Dr Samuel King Hutton remarked: *"Some diseases common in Europe have not come under my notice during a prolonged and careful survey of the health of the* [Labrador] *Eskimos. Of these diseases, the most striking is cancer."*[215]

Remarking on his interview with Joseph Herman Romig, dubbed 'Alaska's most famous doctor', Dr Weston A Price claims that *"...in his* [Romig's] *thirty-six years of contact with these people, he had never seen a case of malignant disease among the truly primitive Eskimos and Indians, although it frequently occurs when they are modernized."*[216]

Dr. Manuel Navarro of Santo Tomas University of Manila, was a world-famed oncologist who was also an early Laetrile clinical pioneer. *"By 1977 he had linked the low incidence of cancer in the native populations of Mindanao* [the Philippines] *to the continual ingestion of many sources of Vitamin B17. That rate, about 1 per 100,000* [less than 1% of the US cancer rate]*, is even smaller than the low rate of cancer in the non-urban Filipino north, where generations of Filipinos have subsisted on* [nitriloside-rich] *cassava, wild rice, wild beans, berries and fruits of all kinds."*[217]

In a letter to Dean Burk, pro-Laetrile head at that time of the Cytochemistry Dept. of the National Cancer Institute, Krebs wrote concerning the North American Indians: *"I have analyzed from historical and anthropological records the nitriloside content of the diets of... various North American tribes.... Some of these tribes would ingest over 8,000 mg of vitamin B17 (nitriloside) a day. My data on the Modoc Indians are particularly complete."*[218]

---

[214] Jones, Rev Livingston French *A Study of the Thlingets of Alaska*, New York, 1914

[215] Hutton, Samuel King *Among the Eskimos of Labrador,* London and Philadelphia 1912

[216] Price, Weston A *Nutrition and Physical Degeneration*, London and New York, 1939

[217] Culbert, M, *What the Medical Establishment Won't Tell You*, ibid.

[218] Griffin, G.Edward, *World Without Cancer*, ibid.

As an example of the low cancer incidence among Indians eating their high 'B17' native diet, Krebs cited a report on the Navajo-Hopi Indians from the *Journal of the American Medical Association* (JAMA), 5th Febuary 1949: *"...the doctors wondered if* [the Indians' diet] *had anything to do with the fact that only 36 cases of malignant cancer were found out of 30,000 admissions to Ganado, Arizona Mission Hospital... In the same population of white persons, the doctors said that would have been about 1,800."*[219]

These stories seem to be the same wherever non-Westernised tribes are encountered. Lack of degenerative diseases in these indigenous tribes led famous explorer Roald Amundsen to comment in 1908:

"My sincerest wishes for our friends the Nechilli Eskimos is, that civilization may never *reach them."*[220]

The *Ecologist* magazine reports:

"Sir Robert McCarrison, a surgeon in the Indian Health Service, observed "a total absence of all diseases during the time I spent in the Hunza valley [seven years]... *During the period of my association with these peoples, I never saw a case of... cancer."*[221]

Dr Alexander Berglas sums up his own findings:

"Civilization is, in terms of cancer, a juggernaut that cannot be stopped... It is the nature and essence of industrial civilization to be toxic in every sense... We are faced with the grim prospect that the advance of cancer and of civilization parallel each other."[222]

Berglas' findings were of course to be corroborated by the World Health Organisation GNP/cancer incidence statistics we looked at

---

[219] Griffin, G Edward *Private Papers Pertaining to Laetrile*, Westlake Village, CA: American Media, 1997, p.13; also Berglas, Alexander, *Cancer Cause and Cure*, ibid.
[220] Amundsen, Roald *The Northwest Passage*, London and New York, 1908
[221] *The Ecologist,* Vol. 28, No. 2, March/April 1998, p. 95
[222] Berglas, Alexander, ibid.

earlier. The common denominator in each of the above cases contributing to a cancer-free society was a lack of toxic, industrialised environment and a natural diet rich in minerals and the nitrilosides.

The other main factor influencing many of the health disasters afflicting the West today centres around our rabid consumption of protein and the way we culturally combine proteins and carbohydrates. As we learned earlier, according to research[223], a diet rich in animal proteins robs our body of its vital supplies of pancreatic enzymes, which are used by the body to terminate healing processes once they are completed.[224] These enzymes are employed during the complicated process the body undergoes as these foreign proteins are broken down into their constituent amino acids and reconstructed as human proteins – a process that is extremely taxing on the body's resources.

Our society has bought into the fear of dying through lack of protein, most believing that unless we chew down meats by the rack-load, we are in serious danger of becoming protein-deficient. This dangerous nonsense came from initial trials conducted on rats. Later it was determined that rats require up to ten times more protein than humans, as evidenced by the commensurate increase in rat mothers' proteins in milk as compared with the protein content of human milk. Today, it is recognised that human protein requirements are not nearly as great as formerly assumed. Nevertheless, the protein trend has been hard to exorcise from the minds of the laity, which in turn has led to an overabundance of serious illnesses and scourges in the West, as Dr Ethel Nelson points out:

"Some of today's most prevalent and devastating diseases in the United States have now been credited to excessive consumption of meat and animal products (milk, cheese, eggs, etc.) and insufficient ingestion of plant foods. These conditions include the so-called "Western diseases": coronary heart disease, diabetes, obesity, appendicitis, diverticulosis of the colon, hiatus hernia,

---

[223] *Cancer Control Journal,* Vol. 6. No.1-6
[224] Binzel, P E, ibid.

hemorrhoids, varicose veins, cancer, osteoporosis, kidney disorders and accelerated sexual development in children." [225]

These diseases, relatively rare in the 1930s, are now found in ever increasing abundance among the 'well-fed' populations of the West. But research shows that ancient populations were also cursed with the diseases that came from heavy meat consumption. In Exodus 15:26 of the Bible, we read:

"If you diligently heed the voice of the Lord your God and do what is right in His sight, give ear to His commandments and keep all His statutes, I will put none of the diseases on you which I have brought on the Egyptians."

What were these diseases of the Egyptians? For that answer, we go to Dr Marc Armand Ruffer, a paleopathologist who, along with his associates, has performed over 36,000 autopsies on Egyptian mummified remains of Pharaonic royals. Ruffer's research demonstrates that most of the diseases striking the Egyptian royalty bear an uncanny resemblance to those killing us today: atherosclerosis (hardening of the arteries), heart disease, cancer, osteoporosis, obesity, tooth decay, arthritis, diverticulosis of the colon, and early sexual development in children. That these diseases were, in the main, being caused by excessive meat eating and wayward diets has since been borne out by further biochemical studies. [226]

In 1992, heart disease alone was claiming 3,000 Americans *a day.* Colon and rectal cancers, now the second cause of cancer death in America, for years have been associated with high-animal-fat, low-fibre diets. Excessive bile acids are required to process high animal fats in the bowel and bile acids are carcinogenic to humans. [227] The transit time for foods through the alimentary tract is prolonged with low-fibre bowel content, allowing a longer period of time for

---

[225] **Nelson MD, Ethel** *The Eden Diet and Modern Nutritional Research*, Twin Cities Conference 1992, Northwestern College, MN, USA.
[226] *Mysteries of the Mummies*, Loma Linda: Slide-tape program produced by Loma Linda University School of Health, 1984
[227] **Galloway, D** *Experimental colorectal cancer: The relationship of diet and faecal bile acid concentration to tumour induction.* Br. J. Surg. 73:233-237, 1986

bile acids to act on bowel mucosa. High pork, beef and chicken consumption correlates closely with the incidence of colon cancer.[228]

Interestingly, Americans have two and a half times the incidence of colon cancer deaths as the Chinese, and yet Chinese-American women who adopt the high-fat, high-meat dietary habits of the United States suffer *four times* the rate of colon cancer as their counterparts in China. In Chinese-American males, the colorectal cancer rate is *seven times* that of their Chinese counterparts. Colon and rectal cancers increase more than 400% among sedentary people, which also correlates with the increased incidence of constipation in this group.[229]

High animal-fat diets have also been linked to breast cancer since high estrogen levels are a predominant factor in breast cancers. Meat-eating women have higher levels of estrogen in the urine than vegetarian women, according to research.[230]

All of which goes to show that there are some serious problems with Western diets that are still not being addressed. Heart disease and cancer, described by experts as being *preventable*, are the two leading killers in the Western world today.

Digestion is the single most strenuous activity our bodies undergo, which is why, after one of our cultural 'heart-attack-on-a-plate' breakfasts, we feel like we are walking on the surface of Jupiter. Excessive meat consumption, coupled with bad food combining of proteins and starches, is also the reason why man is the only creature on Earth that has to process its food using medication – antacids! Other creatures do not improperly combine their foods. As Harvey Diamond, author of *Fit For Life*, wryly remarks, you

---

[228] **Berg, J** Quoted in **Robbins, J** *Diet for a New America*, Stillpoint Publ. 1987. p.254

[229] **Whittemore, A** *Diet, physical activity and colorectal cancer among Chinese in North America and China*, J Natl. Cancer Inst. 82:915-926, 1990. Also Nelson MD, Ethel, ibid.

[230] Schultz, T "Nutrient intake and hormonal status of premenopausal vegetarian Seventh Day Adventist and premenopausal non-vegetarians", *Nutr. Cancer* 4:247-259, 1983

almost never see a lion eating a zebra and having a baked potato with it.

But pick up any menu in a Western restaurant today, and you will see that the majority of items on offer in the starter and main course sections consist of improperly combined proteins and carbohydrates – and mostly cooked to destroy many of the nutrients, *including enzymes*. Steak and fries, chicken and pasta, eggs on toast... the list of woes is as endless as the problems these combinations cause. Because the body produces acids to digest proteins and alkalis for carbohydrates, the two types of juices neutralise each other, eventually producing a rotting mass, parts of which in some cases can still be putrefying inside us up to 70 hours later and may remain with us indefinitely in the form of colonic mucoid plaque. This digestive gridlock produces toxic by-products that get filed around the body and will stay in our systems until we detoxify – which again we almost never do as this is culturally not practised in our society today. On the other hand, proper food combining avoids this build-up and assists in detoxifying our systems from food abuse.

The full science of Natural Hygiene is a fascinating and satisfying study for each of us to make, but unfortunately beyond the scope of this report.[231] One word on properly consuming fruit however. It has been found that the body's elimination (detoxification) cycle runs from approximately 4am to 12 noon in a normal, clock-adjusted body. This is the reason why we awaken with 'fur' on our tongues, bear's breath on the sheets and a desire to go to the bathroom that won't quit. This is our body's time for shedding unwanted weight, ridding the system of toxic by-products and getting the human re-booted for the coming day.

But what do we do to disrupt this natural cycle? Four stacks of Aunt Lily's Arkansas pancakes and syrup go down the hatch during our cultural breakfast (the one we tell everyone we can't do without), or the British variation which is something like: two fried eggs, toast,

---

[231] For a fuller explanation of Natural Hygiene and the concepts and diets that go along with it, please see Day, Phillip *Health Wars*, Credence, 2001; also Day, Phillip *Food For Thought*, Credence, 2001 (both available through www.credence.org)

sausages, bacon, tomatoes, washed down with coffee, followed up by a cigarette or two and the *Sun* newspaper.

More toxic gridlock results. But the worse thing is, the body is prevented from allocating its resources to shedding weight and cleaning itself out, which is essentially the same as detoxifying all the gunk that later gets layered onto the insides of our colons and elsewhere around our bodies. Other methods the body can use to get stuff out of the system are similarly compromised by our culture, like for instance our habit of firing aluminium-laced anti-perspirants directly into our lymph-nodes, jamming them up with an element that has long been linked to the raging incidence of Alzheimer's Disease. Toxins that can't escape this way will inevitably contaminate the lymph and the breast, causing problems down the road when damage occurs and healing processes commence. Then we scrape the fur off our tongues using toothpastes laced with the main constituent of rat poison (sodium fluoride) and rinse our mouths out with water containing chlorine and highly toxic hexafluorosilicic acid, the 'fluoride' with which our governments contaminate our water supplies, which is the toxic waste product taken from phosphate fertilizer pollution scrubbers.

Fruit is an ideal way to detoxify the gunk in our systems during the morning elimination cycle. A fat person is simply someone who has not allowed his or her body to detoxify. Yes, overweight and obesity generally arise as a result of what we have put into our bodies, but our continued overweight and unhealthy condition exists because we are not allowing our system to take out the garbage because we jam up our bodies further with our cultural peccadilloes, like the big breakfast.

Ideally fruit should always be consumed ALONE ON AN EMPTY STOMACH. *Ideally too, the only thing you should consume from the time you arise to lunch-time should be fruit.* Try an experiment for a month and toss out the big breakfast in favour of eating nothing but pieces of fruit in the mornings. The panic clouding your features at this moment at the thought of having to go without the usual breakfast bulk will be off-set with the pleasurable knowledge that your hunger pangs will soon depart once your blood sugar levels regulate your cravings. If it helps, promise yourself the usual heart-attack-on-a-plate if you do not feel satisfied thirty minutes after eating all the fruit you wish to eat. Pineapple, grapes, peaches, oranges, apples, pears (of course, eat the seeds too where appropriate) are all the best kit to get into the kitchen for this great little experiment.

Then when you get to lunch, have lunch! But combine proteins with high water-content vegetables or salad, not with pasta, potatoes, or similar carbohydrates. There's nothing wrong with carbohydrates in their proper whole-food forms, just don't combine them with proteins in the same meal. CUT WAY DOWN ON THE PROTEINS. Vegetables and salad ideally should be enjoyed as close to their native forms (raw and unadulterated) as you can manage. Organic produce is best, uncontaminated with pesticides and other problems we will examine a little later.[232]

Three things will start to happen almost immediately you commence this regimen: firstly, the world will fall out of your tail-pipe. This is your body finally beginning to send the garbage packing. It's all a bit of a mess, but it's leaving – and that's the good news. Loose stools produced from this eating regimen are by no means unhealthy and should be encouraged with as much fruit (on an empty stomach in the morning), high water-content veggies (later in the day) and reasonable exercise as you can manage. A period of gas and bloat will inevitably result as faecal matter and detritus become stirred up. Secondly, You will begin to experience a satisfying return of energy and well-being. Thirdly, you will experience a rapid and steady weight-loss as you proceed with eating your food the way the body likes to process it.

Regular stool-passing is a sign that everything is on the move again. No more 'troubled interactions with nourishment', as the psychologists put it. A new 'you' is emerging as you detoxify. Your skin will appear fresher and healthier looking, your eyes will look clearer, you will sleep better, you will walk funny for a few days until the loose stools firm up again, but MOST IMPORTANTLY, your body has been given back its driver's licence and is now in the

---

[232] Day, Phillip *Food For Thought*, ibid.

hot-seat correctly processing the body's tasks when it should, how it should and why it should.

After four weeks of this experiment, go back and try to eat the heart-attack-on-a-plate for breakfast. You will feel like you have just swallowed the state of Montana, mountains 'n all. And you won't want to do it again.

Another important point is water. Once again traditional medicine believes water is largely nothing more than an inert solvent the body uses to transport the soluent (minerals, proteins, enzymes, etc.) around the body. Yet water is far from inert. The blood is made up of a large percentage of watery serum. Our cells literally owe their life to an adequate supply of fresh, clean water. When the body does not receive a constant, reliable supply of water, it has to ration what's available and cut back on certain functions in order to make the supply go round. Essential systems like the brain are prioritised, others are impaired or cut back until the brain has decided a reliable source of water has been garnered.

Here's the rub. Most citizens have become CHRONICALLY AND DANGEROUSLY DEHYDRATED (especially the elderly), since we decided water was too bland to drink and axed it in favour of beer, wine, sodas, flavoured water and other chemical-laced water alternatives. This has proven a disastrous and dangerous move for the body and society's health in general, and we have been reaping the whirlwind in terms of disease and death as a result. Many doctors today are not trained readily to identify the many water-deficient diseases and associated pains, and so the inevitable prescribing of drugs to treat the symptoms usually results.

The body needs in excess of four pints of water daily (2 litres). Water is used by the body for digestion, detoxifying cells, watering the lungs, keeping the body alkalised and a host of cleaning duties. Water expert Dr Fereydoon Batmanghelidj maintains that asthmas, allergies, diabetes, arthritis, angina, stomach upsets, chronic intestinal complaints and certain other degenerative illnesses are the body's many cries for water, complaints which are dramatically improved with a consistent and long-term intake of fresh, clean water.[233] Dr Batman's best-selling book has helped thousands quash long-term health problems effortlessly and inexpensively. Coffee, tea, diet sodas, beer and a host of other liquids do not qualify as 'clean, fresh water' for the body and should not be consumed by the cancer patient. Many of these are diuretic (water expelling) in their effect because of their chemical compositions. Cancer patients especially should be consuming 4 pints of water a day[234] as part of their intake of vital nutrients, provided they do not have any renal (kidney) damage or disease that will cause complications with urine production resulting from the intake of additional water. Flushing the body with CONSISTENT, long-term water consumption is a superb way to assist with detoxification and hydration and is especially important for cancer patients. Drink a glass half an hour before a meal and then two glasses around two and a half hours afterwards for optimal digestive effects.[235] The remainder of the day's intake of water can be throughout the day.

An indication of dehydration is if the urine is thick, dark yellow and rank in smell. Here the body is cutting back on water usage throughout its various systems due to a chronic shortage.[236] The resultant urine the kidneys make is thus thick with waste consisting of less water than normal, giving rise to a more concentrated urine solution. The body can take several weeks to use water to full effect, so ensure that this vital health bonus is used consistently and effectively. Dr Batman's book is a must for EVERYONE to find out about this incredible and FREE treatment and boon to their health.

Creating your own toxin-free environment too begins and ends with INDIVIDUAL common sense. As Mr Industry, Mrs Corporate

---

[233] Batmanghelidj, F *Your Body's Many Cries For Water*, Tagman Press, 2000 (available at www.credence.org)

[234] A carbon filter attached to a tap/faucet is adequate for producing chlorine- and soluent-free water to drink. This is preferable to plastic-bottled water which can be contaminated with chemicals from the plastic. Water in glass bottles is fine. Patients with kidney complaints should consult their practitioner prior to increasing their consumption of water.

[235] For heartburn, drink water! Every time you feel the pain starting, drink some water. The symptoms usually pass within a few minutes. Constipation too is a sure sign of water starvation, as the body's intestinal peristaltic action extracts every precious drop of water from your food to save losing it, creating gridlock.

[236] Note that B vitamin intakes can also darken the urine.

Drug-Healthcare and Nanny Government are not likely ride in to rescue us any time soon, you, Mrs Smith... you, Mr Williams... you, young Robert... and you, grandma, are going to have to do it for yourselves. Because the food supplies these days are largely depleted of their natural mineral content, supplementation of highly absorbable vitamins, minerals and antioxidants needs to happen in your household, and we're going to come back to this important subject a little later on.

But as we have seen, diets need to change immediately. Suppliers of organically grown fruits and vegetables need to be ferreted out and used henceforth, albeit at greater expense, as our primary food source. There's another irony in this whole bag of potatoes. Natural food is costing more because it isn't pumped full of preservatives and so doesn't last as long in the stores. But, as you will discover, a messy miracle starts to happen when you eat good, clean and wholesome, high-water-content fruits and veggies AND CUT WAY DOWN ON THE MEAT AND OTHER PROTEINS (do you think I have emphasised this enough yet?!). Your body will begin detoxifying the garbage and dropping needless weight at a splendid rate and you feel the benefits of it almost immediately.

I want you to obtain a copy of my book *Health Wars* for a fuller treatment on this great subject of Natural Hygiene.[237] *Health Wars* also has a companion recipe book you can get called *Food For Thought*. These books come with a whole wealth of research and well-grounded common sense for detoxifying your system and getting back to eating basics. These books are not about some magic new special diet. I concentrate on a natural, Hunza-like approach to putting the right gas back in your machine and helping you to re-take control of your own nutrition and healthcare. *Health Wars* will explain more about the simple Natural Hygiene program, the pitfalls of what has happened to our diets and how immediately we can start to put things right.

---

[237] Day, Phillip *Health Wars*, Credence Publications 2001

ACID AND ALKALI ASHES

Q: If we're so rich and smart, how come we're so sick and tired?
A: Because our bodies in the Western world are in a constant state of acid siege.

Dr Ted Morter Jr. has spent a lifetime analysing the effects different foods have on our internal environment. Morter states that the body responds perfectly to every stimulus that is applied to it and each of these body responses is geared towards one aim and one aim only - survival. Sometimes this response is termed 'disease', if it goes against our ideal of what 'health' should be. Morter confirms the fact that the human body likes to dwell in a slight alkali (around pH 7.4). When we acidify our internal environment with certain types of food, the body is forced to neutralise, or buffer this acid using a number of ingenious systems, mostly comprising alkalising minerals, such as sodium, calcium, potassium, magnesium and iron. Urine pH is not necessarily crucial, but blood pH most definitely is. Blood pH must ALWAYS be between 7.35 and 7.45, or else life ends abruptly within a matter of hours.[238]

Foods we eat leave an 'ash' in our system. Rather than the dry flaky stuff that gets all over the carpet when we blow on an old fire, food residues in the body can be solid or liquid, but the 'ash', or residue they leave can either be acid or alkali (and on the odd occasion, neutral). The main acid generators are proteins, whether derived from animal or other sources. The key problem of course is the high level of proteins humans have been persuaded to eat today.

THE DANGERS OF EXCESSIVE PROTEIN
There is nothing wrong with protein. The body needs it, and we'd all be in a disaster situation without it. But the human body does not need anywhere near the level most have been conned into consuming. By the way, notice that the main acid-ash-producing foods are all backed by tremendously powerful and wealthy food

---

[238] Natural (physiological) acid produced through normal cell respiration is easily expelled in the breath via the lungs. Our blood pH is normally 7.35 when it is carting this acid, in the form of carbon dioxide, to the lungs for elimination. Blood is pH 7.45 after it has been 'cleaned up', the CO_2 removed, and then oxygen is taken on to deliver to your heart and the rest of your body.

lobbies with huge advertising budgets – i.e. meat, sugar, grains, coffee, dairy... and yes, even orange juice! A quick survey of the TV content of one evening will give you a picture of how many advertising dollars go into persuading the public to become acidic. Where's the alkali lobby for fruits and veggies? There's no big money in these foods in comparison to the previous list, so there is no lobby.

The protein levels most of us eat today are many times greater than the body actually needs (between 20-30 g a day are the estimated requirements) and the excess we consume can quite literally kill us. Some of us are slogging down up to 10 times the body's protein requirements and more, in our efforts to consume a herd of wildebeest and drink a swimming pool full of milk with our grain 'cereals' laced with refined sugar every morning. How our systems eventually exhaust themselves and collapse with all the acid generated is a book all on its own. But for our purposes here, the key is in understanding the effects of excess protein consumption and how the body tries to deal with it. When the digestive system is hit with a storm of acid derived from excessive protein food metabolism, this acid is potentially lethal and our hard-working body needs to sort the problem in a hurry.

Firstly the brain mobilises mineral buffers to raise the acidic pH of our internal environment towards neutral in an effort to counteract the protein acids.[239] After wolfing down burgers, chicken, eggs, pasta, cheese, seafood, grains – all accompanied by the inevitable acid-producing coffee, tea, sodas and alcohol, the mineral buffers use alkalising minerals and water to combine with the acid generated by these food ashes to raise their pH, before escorting them out of the body via the kidneys. Notice the body loses these alkalising minerals when they are eliminated along with the acid.

THE AMMONIA BUFFER

More often than not, the mineral buffers alone are not strong enough to render the internal environment alkaline enough not to hurt or even damage the kidneys. Fortunately the body has several

---

[239] The pH (potential of hydrogen) scale runs between 0 for pure acid and 14 for pure alkali. 7 is neutral.

back-up systems. The one we're interested in is the ammonia buffer. The kidneys begin producing ammonia, a strong alkali (pH around 9.25), which dramatically raises the pH of the excreta, sometimes as high as pH 8.5. Some people will notice that their urine smells of ammonia, and urinating can even hurt, due to the caustic nature of the solution being squirted out. Hence the need for our old friend, cranberry juice – an acid – which will then normalise the solution and eliminate the pain (there must be an easier way than all this!).

A strong smell of ammonia in the urine may indicate that the body's reserves of alkalising minerals are severely depleted. The body of course can mobilise further supplies of alkalising minerals like calcium, sodium and magnesium, but you won't be happy with where it takes them from (calcium from the bones, etc.). A chronically acidic environment over many years will cause a severe depletion of minerals from the body, resulting in dangers of kidney exhaustion (too much ammonia production and acid damage), osteoporosis, mineral deficiency diseases, and then the auto-immune problems brought on by excess acid lodged in the joints and cartilage, such as arthritis and a host of other complaints.[240] Notice that the body is amoral in this regard. Morter sums up the body's attitude very succinctly:

"Your body doesn't care if you are sick or healthy. It doesn't plan for the future. Your body doesn't think and it doesn't judge. It doesn't care if you are hurting or if you are happy. All it does is respond to survive. Your body makes thousands of perfect survival responses every instant of your life. You may like the results of these responses and call it 'health'. Or you may not like the results and call it 'ill-health'. Your body doesn't care whether you like the responses or not. Survival of this instant is your body's only goal. Not survival later today, or next week, or next year. Survival now. Your body was designed to survive. It wasn't designed to be sick or

---

[240] Kidney dialysis is used when the kidneys can no longer filter out waste products from the body. Without dialysis for damaged kidneys, the body would become overwhelmed with acid and soon die.

well. What it is will be the accumulation of stresses that have been imposed upon it." [241]

Osteoporosis, heart disease, cancer, arthritis, diabetes and other ailments <u>can all be traced to the body's attempts to survive</u>. They can also all be traced to an inherent deficiency in the raw materials (vitamins and minerals) required to get the survival job done. In the context of this book, we've seen that cancer is a healing process that hasn't terminated upon completion of its task, due to malnutrition. External (or internal) damage done to the body will always provoke a response. When we detect the nature of that response, we may exclaim, "Ah, a symptom!" But as Morter declares, the body doesn't care whether you like the results of its survival efforts or not. When you eat, drink, breathe, exercise, rest and think, you elicit a response from your body. So 'health' and 'disease' can be termed effects of your body's responses. Diarrhoea, vomiting, colds, flu, arthritis, osteoporosis and diabetes may not be anyone's idea of a good time, but these dramatic conditions are the result of the body's response to a stimulus or stimuli. As Morter says, if you don't like the body's response, change the stimulus.

ACIDOSIS

With this in mind, we can begin to join a few dots. If the body likes to be alkali, and we are eating extremely acidic (processed), malnourished diets because we are told to by our TV, our body's response will be to buffer the resultant acidic gunk and excrete it rapidly. There are many 'diseases', or body responses, that can be evident from the body accomplishing these actions. Heartburn (acid reflux), indigestion, diarrhoea, mineral loss, resulting in mineral deficiency diseases. Calcium loss diseases, magnesium loss diseases, and so on.

And then, because we are chronically dehydrated because we don't drink water and eat high-water-content food any more (out of fashion), we are plagued by water deficiency ailments, such as constipation, asthma, heartburn, colitis and more ailments than I've got time to write down for you. In addition, your cells really don't go a bundle on being chronically bathed in acid, either inside

---

[241] Morter, M T *An Apple a Day?* BEST Research, Inc. 1997

or outside the cell environment, so there is a potassium buffer response within your cells to raise the pH of your intercellular environment. Cells break down as part of the life and death processes going on in your body all the time, so they add their catabolic acid to the sludge of the fast-food nightmare. Now your brain is forced to order the kidneys to excrete more ammonia to alkalise the excreta before the latter's acid begins burning up the delicate tissues of the kidneys, urethra and other components.

By this time, we've normally managed to scoot down to the doctor's waiting room where we can expect to get drugs, which will 'make us feel better' (they treat the symptoms – not cure the underlying cause). GPs are generally unaware of the alkali/acid struggle going on with many diseases, and they are certainly unaware of the nutrition causation, because most of them haven't been trained in nutrition. Drugs given to a patient will themselves elicit their own responses from the body (side-effects), almost all of which will be acidic. High sugar sodas will fool our body into producing acids in preparation to digest a meal that never arrives, so there is even more acid flying around.

Clinical urine analysis is always useful in providing an indicator of what is going on in the body. When I was living in Los Angeles, there was a big thing going on in the tabloids about how freelance reporters were going through the trash of the stars who lived in Beverly Hills and on Mulholland Drive in order to find material for a 'good' story. While I do not condone in the least this sort of behaviour, going through your body's own trash, using a urine analysis and pH test, yields a lot of useful information. You can learn a lot from the things your body throws away.

A lot of people like to get technical over these issues. They measure protein grams, they measure urine pH, they put themselves through all kinds of strictures, which to me destroy the fun of life. My take is this: simply recognise the signs your body provides that your internal environment is acidic and begin moving it towards alkali by consuming a diet that is 80% alkali-ash-producing foods and 20% of the other stuff. Notice from the lists at the back of the book that almost all fruits and veg are alkali-ash-producing, *and yet many are acidic going in*. Even a humble pear will register pH5.5, and yet pears, along with the malic acid in apples, *have an alkalising effect on the body*. Thus fruits and veggies are the best alkalising tools on the market, containing as they do all the essential minerals the body requires to set up its intricate buffer systems. If your tongue or mouth hurts when you consume fruit, this may be an indicator of how acidic your body is, *before* you begin to do something about it. Start to change your diet gradually using steamed vegetables and your body will appreciate you for your care and gradual education.

ALKALI BODIES ABSORB OXYGEN
Dr Otto Warburg, who received a Nobel Prize in the 1930s, noted that alkaline bodies absorbed up to 20 times more oxygen than acidic bodies. He found that diseased bodies were acidic bodies which repelled oxygen. Warburg worked with almost 50 species of animals and was able to induce cancer in animal tissue simply by acidifying the body and driving out the oxygen.

Warburg found that alkaline bodies are healthy bodies, with a high absorption of life-preserving oxygen. And today, those cultures living long life-spans all have alkalised body systems. The Okinawans, for instance, renowned for their longevity and health, live on their southern Japanese island, which is made predominantly of calcium compounds (coral reef). The water these Japanese citizens consume has been found to contain, per quart, 8,300 mg of dissolved (ionised) calcium and 9,700 mg of un-ionised, non-dissolved calcium for a total of 18 grams of calcium in its various forms. And the Okinawans drink 4/5 quarts a day, and then irrigate their farm soils with it! Researcher Robert Barefoot, who has made a study of the Okinawans, states that by the time he added it up, the Okinawans were getting over 100,000 mg (100g) of calcium in various forms a day and probably violating the RDA over hundredfold for every mineral and vitamin.[242] Yet we are told the RDA for calcium is a miserable 600-1000mg a day.

---

[242] Barefoot, Robert R *The Calcium Factor*, an audio briefing. Available at www.exxelaudio.com; also *The Calcium Factor*, published by Deonna Enterprises Publishing, PO Box 21270, Wickenburg, AZ, 85358, USA

When Otto Warburg explained his exciting acid/alkali conclusions to his medical peers over half a century ago, they threatened to revoke his licence. Yet experiments with ulcerated breast mass and other tumour material show categorically that malignant cells grow prolifically in acid, anaerobic environments, but shrivel and die in calcium- and oxygen-rich alkalis.[243]

Dr Carl Reich, noted nutritional research pioneer, demonstrated that Vitamin D was crucial to the absorption of calcium, and that modern man, in addition to being chronically deficient in ionised calcium, also dwelt mostly under artificial light and was not getting enough interaction of full-spectrum sunlight on the cholesterol in his skin to produce abundant Vitamin D through photosynthesis.

CELLULAR RESPIRATION
Researchers Carafoli and Penniston were studying the calcium ion in the 1980s, and determined that a common trigger exists that precipitates such diverse biochemical processes as the secretion of a hormone and the electrical contraction of a muscle. This trigger, they discovered, was a minute flux of calcium ions. Later research was to show that calcium ions played a far more fundamental role in how each of our cells 'breathes'. Hundreds of research papers today show how cells use an ingenious mechanism of rosette-shaped calcium proteins to open and close ion channels in each cell membrane like doors, which allow nutrients to be taken in and out of the cell.

As the nutrients inside the cell undergo chemical reactions freeing up their nutrient radicals for cell growth, calcium ions are liberated, reducing the pH of this intracellular fluid from 7.4 to around 6.6 and giving it a positive charge. The intracellular and extracellular fluids now have a potential difference, or voltage build-up, of around 70 millivolts. This is enough to bend the calcium rosette 'doors' in the cell membrane open to allow another influx of nutrients into the cell, which react and produce another voltage build-up. In this way, the cell 'breathes', and a continued electrochemical chain reaction ensures a continued production of nutrient raw materials to produce further cells. This entire

---

[243] Barefoot, Robert, ibid.

procedure is completely dependent on ionised calcium being richly abundant in the body and properly absorbed into the bloodstream using the Vitamin D/sunlight catalyst.

Carl Reich, Otto Warburg and later Robert Barefoot understood that calcium has a three-fold effect on vital cell respiration and nutrition:

1. Calcium-bound protein rosettes regulate both the size and the opening and closing of ion 'breathing' channels in every cell wall
2. The calcium ion has the ability to stack nutrients electrically and draw them into the cell through these doors for potential difference (voltage) discharge and chemical reaction
3. Calcium combines with the phosphates in the extracellular and intracellular fluids to create a slightly alkaline, buffered and oxygen-rich medium necessary to sustain life[244]

Gregory R Mundy, Professor and Head of the Division of Endocrinology and Metabolism at the University of Texas, writes as follows:

"A number of important metabolic processes are influenced by small changes in extracellular ionised calcium concentration. These include:

- *The excitability of nerve function and neural transmission*
- *The secretion by cells of proteins and hormones, and other mediators, such as the neurotransmitter acetylcholine[245]*

---

[244] Moolenaar WH, Defize LK & SW Delaat "Calcium in the action of growth factors", *Calcium and the Cell*, Wiley, 1986
[245] Acetylcholine is a neurotransmitter hormone essential for memory. It is formed from the amino acids choline and serine with Vitamin B5, DMAE, pyroglutamate and manganese as co-factor nutrients. An acetylcholine deficiency is being partly blamed for causing Alzheimer's and other memory problem diseases. Key ingredients to mental health are zinc, B5, B6, C, iron and the minerals. In other words, A HEALTHY DIET!

- *The coupling of cell excitation with cell response (for example, contraction in the case of muscle cells, and secretion in the case of secretory cells)*
- *Cell proliferation*
- *Blood coagulation, by acting as a co-factor for the essential enzymes involved in the clotting crusade*
- *Maintenance of the stability and permeability of cell membranes*
- *The mineralisation of newly formed bone"* [246]

Low levels of organic meat (5-10% of the diet) are OK and a source of Vitamins B9 and B12. Meat-eating to excess, aside from causing unwanted and potentially harmful acid toxins, can result in a loss of ionised calcium from the human body. Meat is phosphorus-dominant (an acid), when compared with calcium, which results in calcium phosphates being produced (apatite), which are then precipitated out of the body.

Dr Reich found that when a patient has adequate levels of ionised calcium, his saliva pH range was slightly alkaline at 7.5 to 7.0 (neutral). Body excretions tended to be acidic as the body rids itself of toxins and waste in the ideal way. However, when the body was calcium-deficient, the saliva pH range tended to be acidic, from 6.4 to 4.6, and the body excretions were now alkaline, as the body attempted to mobilise calcium and water to rectify the acid/alkaline balance. Dr James K van Fleet states: *"When the body does not get enough calcium, it will withdraw what little calcium it has from the bones to make sure there is enough in the bloodstream, then the body does its best to bolster the sagging architecture by building bony deposits and spurs to reduce movement and limit activity."* [247] Notice that this is another survival response. Once again, your body does not care whether you hurt or not, it is simply exercising damage control due to an extreme threat situation.

Osteoporosis, arthritis, rheumatism, sclerosis and periodontal disease are all the body's way, not of exhibiting 'disease', but of

---

[246] Mundy, GR "Calcium homeostasis: Hypercalcemia and hypocalcemia", University of Texas
[247] Van Fleet, JK *Magic of Catalytic Health Vitalizers*, Parker Publishing, 1980

discouraging and preventing unnecessary movement during a raging mineral deficiency. Calcium lactates, along with magnesium and Vitamin D, are the sure way to help these symptoms, together with a change of lifestyle and diet.

Alkalising the body in children can happen within days with food and supplements. Adults take much longer, sometimes months, and the elderly may take up to a year to start rendering an alkaline result on the saliva test. The good news is, they will be moving in the right direction if they make some dietary and lifestyle changes for the better.

Want to live to be a healthy hundred? Then find someone who is a healthy hundred, like the Hunzas, and do what they do. Diets low in meat and milk, but rich in 80-85% unrefined plant dietary and alkali ash foods, along with full trace mineral supplementation (including calcium/magnesium/ Vitamin D) are diets rich in mineral-saturated, high-water-content *alkalising* foods that will start combating unnecessary dietary acids and start shifting your body's pH values towards health and longevity – it's as simple as that.

COMMON ALKALI ASH FOODS
(help to control acid in your internal environment)

Almonds
Apples
Apricots
Avocados
Bananas
Beans, dried
Beet greens
Beet
Blackberries
Broccoli
Brussels sprouts
Cabbage
Carrots
Cauliflower
Celery
Chard leaves
Cherries, sour
Cucumbers
Dates, dried
Figs, dried
Grapefruit
Grapes
Green beans
Green peas
Lemons

Lettuce
Milk, goat*
Millet
Molasses
Mushrooms
Muskmelons
Onions
Oranges
Parsnips
Peaches
Pears
Pineapple
Potatoes, sweet
Potatoes, white
Radishes
Raisins
Raspberries
Rutabagas
Sauerkraut
Soy beans, green
Spinach, raw
Strawberries
Tangerines
Tomatoes
Watercress
Watermelon

* Recommended for infants only when mother's milk is not available.
Note: Some of the above foods may seem acidic, but in reality leave an alkali ash in the system.

Convert your diet to 80% alkali ash/ 20% acid ash foods. Ensure that your diet is predominant high-water content foods that are fresh and organic. Supplementation with trace minerals and vitamins is also advised.

COMMON ACID ASH FOODS

Bacon
Barley grain
Beef
Blueberries
Bran, wheat
Bran, oat
Bread, white
Bread, whole wheat
Butter
Carob
Cheese
Chicken
Cod
Corn
Corned beef
Crackers, soda
Cranberries
Currants
Eggs
Flour, white
Flour, whole wheat
Haddock
Lamb
Lentils, dried
Lobster
Milk, cow's ^

Macaroni
Oatmeal
Oysters
Peanut butter
Peanuts
Peas, dried
Pike
Plums ^
Pork
Prunes ^
Rice, brown
Rice, white
Salmon
Sardines
Sausage
Scallops
Shrimp
Spaghetti
Squash, winter
Sunflower seeds
Turkey
Veal
Walnuts
Wheat germ
Yoghurt

^ These foods leave an alkaline ash but have an acidifying effect on the body.

NEUTRAL ASH FOODS THAT
HAVE AN ACIDIFYING EFFECT

Corn oil   Corn syrup   Olive oil   Refined sugar

FORTY FOODS RICH IN VITAMIN B17

Apple seeds
alfalfa sprouts
apricot kernels
bamboo shoots
barley
beet tops
bitter almond
blackberries
boysenberries
brewer's yeast
brown rice
buckwheat
cashews
cherry kernels
cranberries
eucalyptus leaves
currants
fava beans
flax seeds
garbanzo beans
gooseberries

huckleberries
lentils
lima beans
linseed meat
loganberries
macadamia nuts
millet
millet seed
peach kernels
pecans
plum kernels
quince
raspberries
sorghum cane syrup
spinach
sprouts (alfalfa, lentil, mung bean, buckwheat, garbanzo)
strawberries
walnuts
watercress
yams

WHAT IS METABOLIC THERAPY?

Please note: The following information is compiled from treatments carried out by some cancer clinics around the world. These treatments are widely believed by many in the alternative cancer treatment field to be most effective in combating cancers and/or acting as strong cancer preventatives in human and animal systems. No claims are made or implied in providing the following information. The reader must use his discretion and a qualified medical practitioner should always be consulted in the matter of treatment decisions for any cancer.

"If you have cancer, the most important single consideration is to get the maximum amount of Vitamin B17 into your body in the shortest period of time. This is secondary to the medical skill involved in administering it, which is relatively minimal." – Ernst T Krebs Jr

"Metabolic Therapy, put simply, is the use of natural food products and vitamins to prevent and treat cancer by building a strong immune system. The key to stopping the cancer growth doesn't lie in traditional cancer treatments like chemo and radiation therapy or surgery, but in an approach that works with the body instead of against it.

Once the body is cleansed of unnatural substances (detoxification) and vitamins are administered to build the immune system, enzymes are given to begin breaking down the protein shell which surrounds the cancer growth and protects it from the body's immune system. Raw glandular products are also used to augment the body's natural glands. Vitamin B17 (Laetrile) and Vitamin A are then given to the patient to work with the enzymes and immune system to destroy the cancer cell.

Initially Laetrile was looked upon as useless, which it is when used in isolation. However, in Metabolic Therapy, it works with enzymes, vitamins and the immune system to destroy the already weakened cancer." – Dr Harold W Manner

Nutritional therapy for cancer is endorsed by many doctors, including Drs Ernesto and Francisco Contreras, two of the world's most famous and successful cancer physicians. The Contreras Research Team has investigated more than 75 different therapies for cancer in the past 34 years and treated over 100,000 patients. The team continues to seek out the most advanced, effective and compassionate treatments in the world.

B17 METABOLIC THERAPY OVERVIEW
(Phase 1 - The First 21 Days)

The initial phase consists of a 21-day therapy in which clinics include an intravenous drip of B17, sometimes combined with the tissue-penetrating agent DMSO and high doses of Vitamin C. However 500mg amygdalin tablets, together with apricot kernels, are often employed for home use if intravenous treatment is not available. Supplementary therapies in Phase 1 include pancreatic enzyme formula, Vitamin C (up to 10g/day), antioxidants, Vitamins A & E (emulsion), B complex, essential fatty acids, a liquid ionized mineral and vitamin supplement together with actual whole foods that contain B17 (e.g. apricot seeds). Detoxification and full nutritional supplementation procedures are also rigorously followed, along with regular consumption of clean, fresh water (4 pints a day).

B17 METABOLIC THERAPY
(Phase 2 - The Next 3 Months)

The second phase consists of Vitamin B17/amygdalin tablets, apricot seeds, enzymes, Vitamins A, C and E and the continuing detoxification and nutritional procedures initiated in Phase 1.

COMBINED MODALITIES OF TREATMENT

There are no contraindications using amygdalin or any of the components of Metabolic Therapy along with surgery, radiation and chemotherapy, according to the clinics. Surgery, for example, is often life-saving with cancer patients by correcting blockages, repairing fistulas, arresting haemorrhages and removing cancerous growths that are threatening vital organs. If surgery can remove a tumour completely, as in early, non-metastatic cancer, it may conserve the health and save the life of the patient.

WHAT'S IN METABOLIC THERAPY?

Phase 1 Metabolic Pack for the first 21 days

Comes in two alternative forms:

PHASE 1 INTRAVENOUS
With injectable B17/Amygdalin ampoules for administration by qualified medical practitioner. This pack comprises:
- Vitamin B17 ampoules
- Antioxidant capsules
- Pancreatic enzyme tablets
- Vitamin C
- B-Complex
- Vitamin A & E emulsion drops
- Essential fatty acids
- Liquid ionised trace mineral and vitamin supplement
- Hawaiian Noni Juice (anti-tumoural)

Not included is DMSO (dimethyl sulfoxide) for IV administration (some doctors use this compound to achieve fuller penetration of the B17) and apricot kernels.

OR

PHASE 1 ORAL
Injectable/IV Amygdalin is replaced with 500 mg Amygdalin tablets. Otherwise the ORAL Phase 1 includes the same materials as above. Can be purchased for home use. Not included are apricot kernels for nutritional support.

Then, after the first 21 days....

PHASE 2 for the next 3 months

Pack comprises B17 in 500 mg tablet form with the same materials as Phase 1. Not included are apricot kernels for nutritional support.

NUTRITIONAL THERAPY COMPONENT DESCRIPTIONS
(Advanced nutritional elements and their modality)

The following section, compiled by Credence researchers and other contributors, outlines nutritional components that have been studied and used for specific purposes in relation to nutritional support for those who have cancer, or those wishing to exercise prevention. The purpose of this section is to inform and not to recommend any particular course of action or product. Health advice from a qualified health practitioner trained in nutrition is always advised

INJECTABLE B17/LAETRILE/AMYGDALIN
Pharmaceutical grade Vitamin B17 in Metabolic Therapy clinics is administered through injection for the first 21 days (Phase 1) and then orally afterwards (Phase 2). Injectable B17 is also invariably administered together with the tissue penetrating agent dimethylsulfoxide (DMSO) (see DMSO section).

Please note: Clinical tests have repeatedly shown that B17 is only truly effective when used in conjunction with pancreatic enzymes to break down the pericellular coating of the malignant cell.[248] Vitamins A and E in their emulsified form, along with high doses of Vitamin C, are then used in combination with B17 to attack the cancer cell. Clinics administering Metabolic Therapy to their patients always use these or similar supplements.

B17 LAETRILE/AMYGDALIN TABLETS
These pharmaceutical grade tablets contain the active B17 ingredient derived from the kernels of apricots. Usually available in 100 mg or 500 mg tablets. Some people are confused with the terms Laetrile and amygdalin. These names essentially refer to the same compound – Vitamin B17 – and are, to all intents and purposes, interchangeable. These tablets are always taken in conjunction with the apricot seeds. Manufacturers recommend:

---

[248] Manner, HW, Michaelson, TL, and DiSanti, **SJ**. "Enzymatic Analysis of Normal and Malignant Tissues." Presented at the Illinois State Academy of Science, April 1978. Also Manner, HW, Michaelson, TL, and DiSanti, SJ, "Amygdalin, Vitamin A and Enzymes Induced Regression of Murine Mammary Adenocarcinomas", *Journal of Manipulative and Physiological Therapeutics*, Vol 1, No. 4, December 1978. 200 East Roosevelt Road, Lombard, IL 60148 USA

- 2-4 100 mg tablets per day as a nutritional supplement for prevention (apricot seeds have been recommended by doctors in place of tablets for prevention also).
- 4-6 500 mg tablets per day as a nutritional supplement for clinical cancer sufferers, taken in conjunction with enzymes and Vitamins A & E (emulsified).

PANCREATIC ENZYME SUPPLEMENTS
Specific enzymes used in Metabolic Therapy include chymotrypsin (human pancreatic enzyme), trypsin, pancreatin, lipase, amylase, calf thymus (animal enzyme), papain (from papayas) and bromelain (from pineapples). Ernst Krebs also states: *"The demasking effect of these enzymes against the pericellular layer of the malignant cell is something very concrete in the immunology of cancer. Now I prefer, rather than advising the use of bromelain or papaya tablets, that the individual seeking these enzymes get them directly from the fresh ripe pineapple and papaya fruit. As much as half a pineapple a day should be ingested."*

EMULSIFIED VITAMIN A
In 1963 when Dr Contreras initiated his activities as a clinical oncologist, the use of Vitamin A as a useful agent in malignant neoplasm was considered illogical and absurd. Now Vitamin A is accepted as an agent of great use for the major epithelial cancers as well as for epidermis carcinomas, chronic leukaemia and transitional cells.

The first formal studies of the possible anti-tumour effects of Vitamin A were initiated in Germany, by investigators of Mugos Laboratories in Munich. It was a proven fact that lung cancer in Norwegian sailors was less common than in other groups, even though they smoked since childhood. Logic indicated that it had to be the opposite. After studying this phenomenon, it was discovered that they ate abundant quantities of raw fish liver, high in Vitamin A, since childhood. The logical conclusion was that high doses of such a vitamin prevented the growth of lung cancer in heavy smokers. But it was also found that high doses of Vitamin A were toxic, and could cause adverse reactions.

The main focus was to find out how to administer enough Vitamin A to observe preventive or healing effects, without injuring the liver. The solution was found by one of the investigators, when he discovered that unprocessed milk had the vitamin, and children who were breast-fed never experienced toxic effects. Nature had the solution by including Vitamin A in milk in the form of micro-emulsification.

Mugos investigators proceeded to prepare a variety of emulsified concentrations, formulating their famous High Concentration A-Mulsin. One drop contains 15,000 units. They were able to administer over a million units per day in progressive doses, without producing hepatic toxicity. The explanation is that, in emulsified form, Vitamin A is absorbed directly into the lymphatic system without going through the liver in high quantities. Having solved the toxicity problem, it was possible to test the product in high doses. It was demonstrated that emulsified Vitamin A has the following effects:

- In normal doses, it protects epithelium and vision.
- In doses of 100,000 to 300,000 units per day, it works as a potent immune stimulant.
- In doses of 500,000 to 1,000,000 units per day, it works as a potent anti-tumour agent, especially in epidermis and transitional carcinomas.

SHARK CARTILAGE

It has been said that sharks are the healthiest beings on earth. Sharks are immune to practically every disease known to man. Many scientists believe that the shark's skeleton, composed entirely of cartilage, is what is responsible for its incredible immunity to disease.

When administered to cancer patients, shark cartilage has been reported to inhibit the growth of blood vessels, thereby restricting the vitality of the cancerous tumour. In addition, shark cartilage stimulates the production of antibodies and boosts the immune system. Not only is this a non-toxic product recommended for the treatment of cancer, but also for the treatment of inflammatory diseases such as rheumatism and osteoarthritis. Tumours are reported frequently to experience significant reduction in size within one to three months of the initial treatment. It is also noted to enhance the efficacy of Vitamin B17/amygdalin. For in-depth information about shark cartilage, *Jaws of Life* by Dr Alex Duarte and *Sharks Don't Get Cancer* by Dr William Lane provide the complete story. Shark cartilage may be contra-indicated with pregnant or lactating women.

APRICOT SEEDS/KERNELS
Apricot kernels are an inexpensive, rich and natural source of Vitamin B17. They also deliver the vitamins, minerals and enzymes not found in the pharmaceutical derivative of B17.

- ❑ 7 g of seeds per day for life are recommended by Dr Krebs as a nutritional supplement for those exercising cancer prevention. (This equates to 10-12 of the larger kernels or 20-25 of the smaller 'Shalkur' type).
- ❑ 20-28 g of seeds per day are recommended by Dr Krebs as nutritional support for clinical cancer sufferers.

In a minority of cases, cancer sufferers may experience nausea when taking seeds. In this event, clinics recommend that dosage is reduced and then gradually increased as tolerance is gained. Not all apricot seeds are effective. They must have the characteristic bitter taste indicating that the active B17 ingredient is present. Not to be eaten whole. May be pulped, grated or crushed.

Please note: Some cancer sufferers believe that apricot kernels alone are all that is required to fight cancer. Consultation with a qualified health practitioner familiar with Metabolic Therapy is advised for further information. Apricot kernels are usually part of the nutritional support for those exercising cancer prevention *for life* as well as cancer patients undergoing Phase 1 or Phase 2 Metabolic Therapy.

VITAMIN AND MINERAL INTAKES
The huge rise in incidences of cancer and other degenerative diseases is primarily due to the depleted vitamin/mineral content in today's western diet coupled with environmental/chemical toxin factors. The key nutritional ingredients invariably missing for cancer are B17 and the trace mineral selenium. A recent US study showed an overall drop of 50% in cancer deaths and a fall of 37% in new cancer cases, especially lung, bowel and prostate – among 1,300 volunteers taking supplements for four years.[249] Mineral supplementation is most effective in the ionised 'liquid suspension' colloidal form, where an exceptionally high assimilation of the nutrients by the body is expected, as against other forms of minerals, such as the metallic

---

[249] *Daily Mail*, 28th July 1999, p. 31

variety. Our bodies use minerals as raw material. These cannot be manufactured by the body and so have to be present in the food and liquids we ingest. Sadly, as mentioned previously, our food chain is severely depleted of minerals, resulting in over 150 nutritional deficiency diseases that are now striking our societies with increasing intensity.

To combat this very real threat, mineral and vitamin supplementation, far from being a quaint health fad, is essential for everyone and can literally make the difference between life or death, especially for those with cancer.

ANTIOXIDANTS
Scientists tell us that vitamins A, C, and E, as well as beta carotene and other antioxidant bioflavonoids, are vitally important to good health. But there are antioxidant formulae around now that have many more times the power of Vitamin C and Vitamin E. Current theory holds that oxidation elements, or free radicals as they are sometimes known, damage healthy cells when they rob electrons to render themselves stable. Ongoing free-radical activity is dangerous for cancer sufferers. Antioxidants such as Vitamin C neutralise the damage caused by free radicals. The problem is, after having entered the body, most antioxidant molecular structures will grab one free radical and then change into an inert state, ceasing to be of further radical-scavenging value. The additional problem is that even when an antioxidant neutralises a free radical, the process creates an off-shoot free radical that is slightly different and less potent in variety, which in turn creates another, and so on. Typical antioxidants have no ability to address this free radical cascading effect on an ongoing basis.

Thus a constant supply of good antioxidant material is vital to the body and essential both as a staple nutritional support factor for cancer sufferers as well as those who are exercising prevention.

DIMETHYL SULFOXIDE (DMSO)
DMSO is a by-product of the wood and paper industry and has gained prominence in recent times as a highly effective agent in the treatment of herpes, cancer and other diseases. DMSO is a unique solvent that penetrates the blood/brain barrier and is used with B17 intravenously to deliver the principal treatment deep into the body without changing

the latter's chemical structure. DMSO is renowned for its ability to penetrate the body's tissue rapidly and completely. Credence has a special report on DMSO which can be obtained free by e-mailing your request to dmso@credence.org.

VITAMIN C

Dr Linus Pauling, often known as the 'Father of Vitamin C' and twice awarded the Nobel Prize, declared that large intakes of up to 10g of the vitamin each day aids anti-cancer activity within the body. Pauling was largely derided for making these declarations, but today, large doses of Vitamin C are used by many practitioners for cancer patients in nutritional therapy, who believe Pauling was right and that the popular nutrient is indispensable to the body in its fight to regain health from cancer.

Several studies have suggested that Vitamin C may reduce levels of lead in the blood. Epidemiological studies have shown that people with elevated blood serum levels of Vitamin C had lower levels of blood toxicity. An examination of the data from the Third National Health and Nutrition Examination Survey, enrolling 4,213 youths aged 6 to 16 years and 15,365 adults 17 years and older from 1988 to 1994, found a correlation between low serum ascorbic acid levels and elevated blood lead levels. The authors conclude that high ascorbic acid intake may reduce blood lead levels.[250]

An analysis of the Normative Aging Study, which enrolled 747 men aged 49 to 93 years from 1991 to 1995, found that lower dietary intake of Vitamin C may increase lead levels in the blood.[251] A study of 349 African American women enrolled in the project Nutrition, Other Factors, and the Outcome of Pregnancy found that vitamin-mineral supplementation resulted in increased serum levels of ascorbic acid and decreased serum levels of lead. The authors concluded that maternal use of a vitamin supplement with ascorbic acid and vitamin E

---

[250] Simon JA, Hudes ES "Relationship of Ascorbic Acid to Blood Lead Levels." *JAMA.* 1999;281:2289-2293.
[251] Cheng Y, Willett WC, Schwartz J, Sparrow D, Weiss S, Hu H "Relation of nutrition to bone lead and blood lead levels in middle-aged to elderly men. The Normative Aging Study." *Am J Epidemiol* 1998 Jun 15;147(12):1162-1174.

might offer protection from lead contamination of the foetus during pregnancy.[252]

Because smoking lowers levels of ascorbic acid in the body, researchers theorised that Vitamin C supplementation may affect blood lead levels in smokers. A clinical study was performed on 75 adult men 20 to 30 years of age who smoked at least one pack of cigarettes per day, but had no clinical signs of ascorbic acid deficiency or lead toxicity. Subjects were randomly assigned to daily supplementation with placebo, 200 mg of ascorbic acid, or 1000 mg of ascorbic acid. After one week of supplementation, there was an 81% decrease in blood-lead levels in the group taking 1000 mg of ascorbic acid daily.[253]

Dosage recommended by Linus Pauling is up to 10g/day. High levels of Vitamin C however can cause diarrhoea and may be contra-indicated with certain chemotherapy treatments. Check with your physician.

IMPLEMENTING CHANGES – CONVERTING YOUR BATHROOM

As many of the harmful ingredients we examined earlier can be found in the average bathroom, clear these out in one fell swoop and replace with safe and environmentally friendly alternatives (see *Contacts!* for advice on where to obtain these). At the moment, many of us are brushing our teeth with rat poison, washing our hair out with cheap engine degreasants, putting liquid paraffin on our babies in the form of baby oil, firing aluminium into the lymph nodes under our arms and using constituents of brake fluid and antifreeze in our make-up and personal care formulae. Does this make sense?

EXERCISE IN MODERATION

Research shows that those with a sedentary lifestyle are more prone to cancer and heart problems. A moderate exercise program will cleanse the body, get the lymph system moving and active, tone up pieces of the body and generally get everything in proper working order. Simply MOVE! Walking, a non-threatening hour in the gym twice or three

---

[252] West WL, Knight EM, Edwards CH, et al. "Maternal low level lead and pregnancy outcomes." *J Nutr*. 1994 Jun;124(6 Suppl):981S-986S.
[253] Dawson EB, Evans DR, Harris WA, Teter MC, McGanity WJ "The effect of ascorbic acid supplementation on the blood lead levels of smokers." *J Am Coll Nutr*. 1999 Apr;18(2):166-170.

times a week or cycling are ideal and immensely enjoyable once you get on the pro-active program. If you sit still all day long, you might as well not breathe! Life is about healthy action. Celebrate your life by looking, moving and feeling the way your body was designed to be.

THE TOTAL NUTRITIONAL PROGRAM
by Phillip Binzel MD

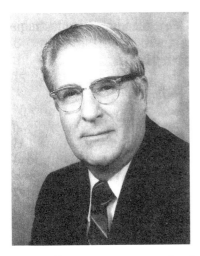

I am going to outline, *in generalities*, the treatment that I use. Please note that patients and their cancers vary considerably and a qualified practitioner should be employed to carry out any treatments – even nutritional ones.

The whole purpose of the nutritional program for cancer is to do two things:

- To put into the body the nutritional ingredients that the body needs in order to allow its immunological defense mechanisms to function normally, and
- To take away from the body those things that are detrimental to the normal function of its immunological defense mechanisms.

There are three parts to this program:

1. Vitamins, minerals and enzymes
2. Nitrilosides
3. Diet

VITAMINS, MINERALS AND ENZYMES
Vitamin and mineral supplement (as directed)
Vitamin C 1 gram – 1 twice daily
Vitamin E 400 IU – 1 twice daily
Enzyme capsules (trypsin, chymotrypsin, bromelain, papain, etc.) 2 three times a day
Pangamic acid (Vitamin B15) 100mg – 1 three times daily
Vitamin A emulsion (25,000 IU Vitamin A per drop) 5 drops daily

Since vitamins are food, they should be taken with meals or immediately afterwards.

224

NITRILOSIDES

In order to supply the necessary nitrilosides, I use Amygdalin (Laetrile). Laetrile is available in 500 mg tablets and in vials (10cc – 3g) for intravenous use. I use both forms. The dosage I use is as follows:

The intravenous Laetrile is given three times weekly for three weeks with at least one day in between injections (Monday, Wednesday and Friday). The Laetrile is not diluted and is given by straight IV push over a period of one to two minutes depending on the amount given.

The dose for the intravenous Laetrile is:

1st dose 1 vial (10cc – 3 g)
2nd Dose 2 vials (20cc – 6 g)
3rd dose 2 vials (200cc – 6 g)
4th through 9th doses 3 vials (30cc – 9 g)

Following this first three weeks of IV injections, the patient then has one injection of 1 vial (10cc – 3 g) once weekly for three months. If the patient notices a considerable difference in the way they feel when the injections are reduced to once weekly, the injections are increased to two or three times a week for three weeks. The dose is then reduced again to once weekly. This is repeated as often as is necessary until the patient notices no difference with the reduced dosage.

The oral Amygdalin (Laetrile) is given in a dosage of 1 gram (two 500 mg tablets) daily on the days on which the patients do not receive the intravenous Laetile. I have them take both tablets at the same time at bedtime on an empty stomach with water. The water is important because there are some enzymes in the fruits and vegetables and in their juices which will destroy part of the potency of the Laetrile tablets while they are in the stomach. Once the stomach has emptied, this is no problem.

It should be noted that I do not start my patients on their Laetrile, either IV or orally, until the patients have been on their support vitamins, minerals, enzymes and diet for a period of ten days to two weeks. I find that the Laetrile seems to have little or no effect until a sufficient quantity of other vitamins and minerals are in the body. Zinc, for example, is the transportation mechanism for the Laetrile. In the absence of sufficient quantities of zinc, the Laetrile will not get into the tissues. The body will not rebuild any tissues without sufficient quantities of Vitamin C, etc.

When I start the intravenous and oral dosages of Laetrile, I also begin to increase the amount of Vitamin C. I have my patients increase their Vitamin C by one gram every third day until they reach of level of at least six grams. In some patients, I use more. I find there are some patients who develop irritation of the stomach or diarrhea with the larger doses of Vitamin C. I find by increasing this by one gram every third day that, if these symptoms develop, I can reduce the Vitamin C to a level that causes no problem. I find that most of my patients tolerate the higher doses of Vitamin C very well.

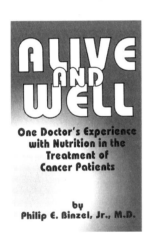

ALIVE AND WELL

One Doctor's Experience with Nutrition in the Treatment of Cancer Patients

by
Philip E. Binzel, Jr., M.D.

On the days that my patients receive intravenous Laetrile, I ask them not to take their Vitamin A. There have been some studies indicating that Vitamin A may interfere with the body's ability to metabolize intravenous Laetrile. This has not been fully proven, but I choose to have my patients not take their Vitamin A drops on the days on which they receive their intravenous Laetrile. Also I tell my patients not to take the Laetrile tablets on the days that they receive the intravenous Laetrile. They have received intravenously as much Laetrile as the body can handle for that period of time. There are no ill-effects from taking the tablets on those days, but the effect of the tablets is wasted.

The level of nitrilosides in the body can be monitored. When the body metabolizes nitrilosides, the by-product is thiocyanate. Thiocyanate levels in the blood can be measured. I find, in general, that the patients who do best are those in whom the thiocyanate is between 1.2 and 2.5 Mg/DL. This level can be raised or lowered by increasing or decreasing the dosage of the Laetrile tablets.

I do not want to leave the impression that Laetrile is the only source of nitrilosides. There are some 1500 foods that contain nitrilosides. These include apricot kernels, peach kernels, grape seeds, blackberries, blueberries, strawberries, bean sprouts, lima beans and macadamia nuts. The advantage of using Laetrile in the cancer patient is that Laetrile is a concentrated form of nitrilosides.

About this Author: Philip Binzel, a native of Bowling Green Kentucky, has been practising medicine for over forty years. He is a graduate of the Medical School at St. Louis University in Missouri and did his internship at Christ Hospital in Cincinnati, Ohio. His experiences with metabolic therapy over many years are accurately described in his book, *Alive and Well*, available through www.credence.org.

IMPORTANCE OF DIET
by Phillip Day

The cancer patient must pay special attention to their diet for the remainder of their life. Many doctors practicing metabolic therapy will modify their patient's diet immediately in the following ways:

No meat, no sugar, no caffeine, no dairy, no eggs, no fish, no white (refined) flour
Reduce intake of citrus fruits
Half a pineapple in the morning
Organic food only
Plenty of clean, fresh water (2-3 liters a day/4-6 pints)
Nutritional supplementation

As Dr Binzel states:

"If it is animal or if it comes from an animal, you cannot have it. If it is not animal or does not come from an animal, you can have it, but you cannot cook it."

The reminder of food available to eat is not as restrictive as people at first realise. Proteins can come from a number of excellent sources, such as whole grains, corn on the cob, buckwheat, nuts, beans (soup beans, split-pea, navy beans, kidney beans, etc.). Food should eaten

227

raw in order not to damage vital enzymes that usually perish at cooking temperatures. The lack of animal proteins in the diet enables the body to utilize pancreatic enzymes to damask the pericellular coating of trophoblast cells.

Frozen foods are also forbidden, as they usually have undergone some form of processing, such as blanching pasteurization or sterilized, killing any available enzymes.

The widest range of raw vegetables (organic) should be consumed. The body takes in its amino acids ideally from high quality vegetation, fruits and nuts. From these aminos we then construct our human proteins accordingly.

For concrete food strategies, please obtain a copy of *Food for Thought* from Credence Publications.

AMERICAN CANCER SOCIETY INDICTED

CHICAGO, 25th Oct 1999 /PRNewswire/ - The following was released today by the Cancer Prevention Coalition:

An article, "American Cancer Society: The World's Wealthiest 'Non-Profit' Institution," by Dr Samuel Epstein, just published in the *International Journal of Health Services*, the leading international public health and policy journal, charges that the American Cancer Society (ACS) *"is fixated on damage control ... diagnosis and treatment ... and basic molecular biology, with indifference or even hostility to cancer prevention."* ACS also trivializes the escalating incidence of cancer which has reached epidemic proportions and makes grossly misleading claims on dramatic progress in the treatment and cure of cancer. This myopic mindset and derelict policy is compounded by interlocking conflicts of interests with the cancer drug, agrichemical, and other industries. The following is illustrative:

- Since 1982, the ACS has adopted a highly restrictive policy insisting on unequivocal human evidence on carcinogenicity before taking any position on cancer risks. Accordingly, the ACS has actively campaigned against the 1958 Delaney law banning the deliberate addition to food of any amount of chemical additive shown to induce cancer, even in well-validated federal animal tests.
- In a joint 1992 statement with the Chlorine Institute, the ACS supported the continued use of organochlorine pesticides in spite of their recognized environmental persistence and carcinogenicity.
- In 1993, just before PBS *Frontline* aired the special entitled "In Our Children's Food," the ACS sent a memorandum in support of the pesticide industry to some 48 regional divisions which pre-emptively trivialized pesticides as a cause of childhood cancer and reassured the public that residues of carcinogenic pesticide in food are safe, even for babies.
- In *Cancer Facts & Figures*, the ACS annual publication designed to provide the public with "basic facts" on cancer, there is little or no mention of prevention. Examples include

no mention of: dusting the genital area with talc as a known cause of ovarian cancer; parental exposure to occupational carcinogens, domestic use of pesticides, or frequent consumption of nitrite colored hot dogs (resultingly contaminated with carcinogenic nitrosamines) as major causes of childhood cancer; and prolonged use of oral contraceptives or hormonal replacement therapy as major causes of breast cancer. Facts & Figures, 1997, also misrepresented that *"since women may not be able to alter their personal risk factors, the best opportunity for reducing mortality is early detection."* This statement ignores overwhelming evidence on a wide range of ways by which women of all ages can reduce their risks of breast cancer, including regular use of the cheap non-prescription and safe drug aspirin.

♦ The ACS, together with the National Cancer Institute, has strongly promoted the use of Tamoxifen, the world's top-selling cancer drug, ($400 million annually) manufactured by Zeneca, for allegedly preventing breast cancer in healthy women, evidence for which is highly arguable at best. More seriously, ACS has trivialized the dangerous and sometimes lethal complications of Tamoxifen including blood clots, lung embolism, and aggressive uterine cancer, and fails to warn that the drug is a highly potent liver carcinogen.

Conflicts of interest are further reflected in the ACS Foundation Board of Trustees, which includes corporate executives from the pharmaceutical, cancer drug, investment, and media industries. They include David R. Bethume, president of Lederle Laboratories, Gordon Binder, CEO of Amgen (a leading biotech cancer drug company), and Sumner M. Redstone, chairman of the Board of Viacom, Inc.

Other concerns relate to the "non-profit status" of the ACS whose annual budget is some $500 million. Most funds raised go to pay high overhead, salaries, fringe benefits, and travel expenses of national executives in Atlanta, CEO's who earn six-figure salaries in several states, and hundreds of other employees working in some 3,000 regional offices. Less than 16% of all monies raised are spent on direct patient services; salaries and overhead for most ACS affiliates exceed 50%, although most direct community services are handled by unpaid volunteers. While ACS cash assets and reserves approach $1 billion, it continues to plead poverty and lament the lack of funds for cancer research. Not surprisingly, the Chronicle of Philanthropy, the leading U.S. charity watchdog, has concluded that the ACS is "more interested in accumulating wealth than saving lives." It should further be noted that the ACS uses 10 employees and spends $1 million a year on direct lobbying, and is the only known charity that makes contributions to political parties.

Based on these considerations the International Journal of Heath Services article urged that, in the absence of drastic reforms, contributions to the ACS should be diverted to public interest and environmental groups directly involved in cancer prevention. This is the only message that this "charity" can no longer ignore.

ABOUT THIS AUTHOR

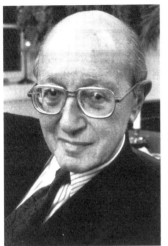

Samuel Epstein MD is a world-renowned authority on the causes and prevention of cancer. He was named the 1998 winner of the Right Livelihood Award (also known as the 'Alternative Nobel Prize'). Dr Epstein has devoted the greater part of his life to studying and fighting the causes of cancer. He is Professor of Occupational and Environmental Medicine at the School of Public Health, University of Illinois Medical Center at Chicago, and the chairman of the Cancer Prevention Coalition.

As the author of *The Politics of Cancer* and *The Breast Cancer Prevention Program*, Dr Epstein advocates the use of cosmetics and other products that are free from suspected carcinogens.

THE VITAMIN C 'SCARE'
by Steven Ransom
Credence Research

The following article is reprinted in full from Credence archives. Its findings prove most relevant to the debate on how Big Business, Big Pharma and Big Government are trying to monopolise all sectors of public health through scare tactics and false propaganda.

THEY SAY THAT VITAMIN C
CAN INCREASE THE RISK OF CANCER
Oh yes? And who's 'they'?

VITAMIN C CANCER FEAR - High doses of Vitamin C could increase the risk of cancer, scientists warn today....

So begins the 15th June 2001 UK Daily Mail front-page report, outlining the work of Dr Ian Blair, resident researcher at the University of Pennsylvania Pharmacology Unit. The Mail headline appears to be in direct conflict with Dr Blair's own statement: "Absolutely, for God's sake, don't say Vitamin C causes cancer." (Yahoo News, Thursday, 14th June 2001) But of course, The Mail and others have shamelessly done exactly that. To the less discerning reader, the story raises worrisome questions as to the wisdom of high-level Vitamin C supplementation. If these worldwide headlines have served any useful purpose at all, it has been to confirm the moral/intellectual void currently reigning in today's mass media 'news' departments.

CASTING ASPERSIONS
At a more fundamental level, why is Dr Blair conducting tests on the efficacy of Vitamin C at all? We are about to discover that certain parties have a very definite interest in casting aspersions upon Vitamin C. To our knowledge, the information you are about to read has not been included in any of the latest, and now worldwide **'Vitamin C Cancer Scare'** headlines generated by Dr Blair's findings.

A GOLDEN RULE
Dr Blair postulates that high consumption of Vitamin C (a most beneficial adjunct in non-toxic cancer recovery treatment) might actually cause human tissue degeneration, which in turn could lead to a

heightened risk of contracting cancer. And it is here that we arrive at our first golden rule: when it comes to assessing the veracity of any scientific claim, we must always read between the lines – we must search for what the report does not say. We must especially be on the look-out for that hoary old chestnut, otherwise known as vested interests. A University of Manchester research methodology handbook contains the following valuable advice:

"Science and research must be studied in the context of all the interested parties involved. The questions centre on determining the relative weight of the various allies in the 'fact-creating' process - e.g. funding bodies, businesses, departments of state, professions and other scientists. In analysing scientific debates, one should always ask what social, institutional, political and philosophical interests lie behind often apparently 'neutral' and 'technical' knowledge claims." (University of Manchester Institute of Science & Technology (UMIST) research methodology course handout, 1994)

On the matter of the 'fact creation' process, renowned author John Le Carré recently stated:

"Big Pharma [the industry in general] *is engaged in the deliberate seduction of the medical profession, country by country, worldwide. It is spending a fortune on influencing, hiring and purchasing academic judgment to a point where, in a few years' time, if Big Pharma continues unchecked on its present happy path, unbought medical opinion will be hard to find."* (The Nation, New York, Interview with John Le Carré, 9th April 2001)

BOUGHT?
With the above in mind, let's put Dr Blair's University of Pennsylvania under the spotlight and see what encouragement Dr Blair might have had in taking his extraordinary and apparently misquoted position against Vitamin C. We must ask the following questions: what Big Pharma influences might there be supporting the University of Pennsylvania Cancer Center (UPCC) and its mother ship, the University of Pennsylvania Health Service? What is the relative weight of the funding bodies? If industry sponsorship is taking place, are UPHS personnel free to exercise unbiased, critical thinking? Or are there grounds to suspect that UPHS has been 'bought' - that

somewhere along the line, vested interests have 'purchased academic judgment'? Before tackling the Vitamin C issue itself, the following UPHS general statistics are very revealing.

CERTAIN ALLIANCES

In May 2000, Dr Ian Blair's employers at UPCC received a $26 million, five-year Core Grant from the National Cancer Institute (NCI) - the largest and most influential conventional cancer treatment institution in the world. In fact, UPCC has been continuously funded by the NCI Core Grant mechanism since the grant was created by the National Cancer Act in the early 1970's. Currently, UPCC is awash with more than $100 million in cancer research funding: $37 million is from the National Cancer Institute; $43 million from closely affiliated organisations, such as the National Institutes of Health, the institution which actually funded Dr Blair's Vitamin C research; another $12 million from foundational support such as the American Cancer Society and the Leukaemia Society; and between $8 and $10 million from various pharmaceutical companies. Earlier, in June of 1999, UPCC received a $4.5 million gift from the William H. Gates Foundation to research conventional treatments for non-Hodgkin's lymphoma.

Aside from the Bill and Melinda Gates connection, OncoLink, the University of Pennsylvania Cancer Center, is sponsored very generously by the following corporations: Amgen, the world's largest independent biotechnology company; Aventis, Ortho Biotech, Inc., Varian, Inc., Janssen Pharmaceutica, AstraZeneca, Pharmacia Upjohn and Pfizer. These corporations are very big indeed, and their names represent no mean sponsorship committee.

MORE ALLIANCES

In March 2001, UPHS announced a strategic alliance with Siemens Medical Systems, Inc. Under the terms of the purchasing agreement, UPHS will make an initial discounted purchase of cardiology, radiology and radiation oncology equipment from Siemens, who will also service and maintain the biomedical equipment already in place at designated UPHS sites over the life of the agreement. In the year 2000, Siemens Medical Solutions, based in Iselin, New Jersey, reported new orders of $5.65 billion, sales of $5.44 billion and employs 27,000 worldwide. *"This is the kind of alliance that will be critical in our continuing financial recovery and to assure our position as a leading national health system,"* said Robert D. Martin, Ph.D., Chief Executive Officer of UPHS.

A good relationship with Siemens may well be critical to UPHS' financial recovery, but does this kind of dependent alliance foster the aforementioned necessary climate for critical thinking? What if there are privately held UPHS reservations over the Siemens equipment, methodology or ethos? Who will break rank first? Will anyone? What kind of commercially gagged framework are the UPHS staff now locked into with Siemens?

YET MORE CORPORATE ALLIANCES
On April 26, 2001, UPCC announced a business partnership with Integral PET Associates, the nation's leading operator of fixed-site Positron Emission Tomography (PET) cancer scanners. A patient receiving a PET scan today is injected with a radiopharmaceutical, such as flurodeoxyglucose (FDG), about 45 minutes before the scan, which takes about two hours. The radiopharmaceutical tracer emits signals which are then picked up by the PET scanner.

A computer reassembles the signals into recognisable images to determine if a cancer has spread, if a particular treatment is effective, or if a patient is disease-free. IPA will now be seeking to supply major hospitals throughout Pennsylvania with this very expensive equipment. Installing and operating a PET scanner typically costs around $1,600,000 in up-front capital costs, plus an additional $800,000 in yearly staff and operational costs.

A short visit to the UPHS website at www.med.upenn.edu will not only confirm all of the above information, but will also confirm that these alliances represent only a small percentage of the long-standing conventional 'friendships' UPHS has fostered with Big Pharma over the years. Given the strictly conventional source of sponsorship monies received at UPHS, what chance will the following statements have of being 'allowed' to feature on the UPHS cancer information page?

"If I contracted cancer, I would never go to a standard cancer treatment centre. Cancer victims who live far from such centres have a chance." **Professor Charles Mathe, French cancer specialist**

"...as a chemist trained to interpret data, it is incomprehensible to me that physicians can ignore the clear evidence that chemotherapy does much, much more harm than good." **Alan C Nixon, PhD, former president of the American Chemical Society**

"Doctors are too busy to dig into the statistics of cancer treatments, they assume that what they are taught at school or what is demonstrated in the pages of briefing journals is the best treatment. They cannot afford to suspect that these treatments are only the best for the pharmaceutical companies that influence their 'institutions of higher learning'." **Paul Winter, The Cancell Home Page.**

"To the cancer establishment, a cancer patient is a profit center. The actual clinical and scientific evidence does not support the claims of the cancer industry. Conventional cancer treatments are in place as the law of the land because they pay, not heal, the best. Decades of the politics-of-cancer-as-usual have kept you from knowing this, and will continue to do so unless you wake up to this reality." **Lee Cowden MD**

"Almost every patient treated with IL2 (a current conventional cancer treatment) suffered fever, malaise, nausea or vomiting, diarrhoea, sharp drops in blood pressure, skin rashes, breathing difficulties, liver abnormalities and irregularities in blood chemistry. Rosenberg himself details a number of horrifying case histories, and one in particular where the administration of IL2 had precipitated amongst other things, vomiting, swollen joints, lung fluid and 'vascular leak syndrome' where blood would ooze through the vessel walls and collect under the skin." **Steven Rosenberg, The Transformed Cell, Putnam Press, 1992**

"Dr Linus Pauling, often known as the 'Father of Vitamin C' and twice awarded the Nobel Prize, declared that large intakes of up to 10g of the vitamin each day aids anti-cancer activity within the body. Pauling was largely derided for making these declarations, but today, large doses of Vitamin C are used by many practitioners for cancer patients in nutritional therapy, who believe Pauling was right and that the popular nutrient is indispensable to the body in its fight to

regain health from cancer." **Phillip Day, Cancer, Why We're Still Dying to Know The Truth, Credence Publications, 2001.**

"Do not let either the medical authorities or the politicians mislead you. Find out what the facts are, and make your own decisions about how to live a happy life and how to work for a better world." **Linus Pauling** http://www.cforyourself.com

The above remarks are representative of a vast library of well-sourced contrary information which sensibly questions the validity and efficacy of conventional cancer treatments based on a huge amount of clinical research and data. Naturally, with all these expensive and patented treatments available to fight cancer, the cancer rates should be going down. They are not. They are increasing.

STAGGERING AMOUNTS
UPHS is locked into the conventional cancer framework - a framework which today, rightly stands accused of achieving no measurable success at all in its approach to the treatment of cancer, immense success in causing widespread, unnecessary death through its application of lethal and highly toxic pharma-radiation treatments, and even greater success in rewarding itself absolutely staggering amounts of money in the whole grisly process. That these cancer corporations have become incredibly wealthy through their 'chemo 'til we drop' approach is a fact which Messrs Siemens, Zeneca, Upjohn, Glaxo, Rhône Poulenc cannot deny.

COMMON SENSE
Pauling was right. We have been seriously misled. Taking the Siemens $multi-million technology as an example. It may well detect certain forms of cancer, but upon detecting it, what then happens? Quite simply, a bewildered, obedient, grateful and unsuspecting cancer sufferer is immediately directed towards the door marked 'iatrogenic (doctor-induced) illness and probable death.' Closer examination of today's orthodox cancer treatments clearly reveals that the conventional path is fraught with toxic danger. But the CEO of UPHS has made it quite clear that *'the Siemens alliance* [one of so many] *is critical to the financial security of UPHS'*.

238

This is why we will hear no publicly dissenting voices from UPHS as to the horrific realities associated with 20th and 21st century conventional cancer treatments. The corporate big boys' riches must continue to flow.... and a handsome proportion of it into the coffers of the very dependent UPHS, of course, 'to assist in their financial recovery'.

SO WHY THE SLUR ON VITAMIN C?
As has already been stated, conventional cancer treatment represents a $multi-billion a year industry. These vast profits are fiercely protected by the industry giants. But their treatments in no way address the underlying causes of cancer. Cancer is a nutritional/toxic/environmental condition, which, in a great number of instances, can be successfully reversed through the application of a sound nutritional approach and common-sense lifestyle changes. Linus Pauling, dubbed 'the father of Vitamin C', sensibly promoted the benefits of consuming high doses Vitamin C in the prevention of and battle against cancer.

HALF-TRUTHS AND LIES
So why aren't we hearing about these natural treatment successes? Why aren't they being heralded across the world? The answer is money. Despite the multitudinous successes in cancer regression through nutrition, and through extensive application of vital elements such as Vitamin C, Vitamin B17, pancreatic enzymes and other co-factors, Big Pharma is doing all it can to silence these success stories.

To have it become widely known that cancer can be successfully treated without toxic and profitable pharmaceuticals would be catastrophic for its business. Who would continue to purchase these products? What would the Siemens, Glaxo and Upjohn shareholders have to say about that?

To their shame, vested interests are keeping well-proven, non-toxic cancer treatments from the public domain. This is why, under 'cancer treatments', the UPHS website says this of vitamin B17:

"Several patients displayed symptoms of cyanide poisoning, including muscle weakness and impaired reflexes, or had life-threatening levels of cyanide in their blood. (Laetrile can release cyanide, which is a

highly toxic chemical.) The researchers concluded that Laetrile is not effective as a cancer treatment and is harmful in some cases." [254]

Now read this contrary extract from a radio talk show, featured in Phillip Day's *Cancer, Why We Are Still Dying To Know the Truth:*

Radio host Laurie Lee: *"So this is verified, that Laetrile [B17] can have this positive effect?"*

Dr Ralph Moss: *"We were finding this and yet, we in Public Affairs were told to issue statements to the exact opposite of what we were finding scientifically."*

At the time, Ralph Moss was former Assistant Director of Public Relations at Memorial Sloan Kettering, NY, a leading American conventional cancer research facility.

ONLY A LUNCH AWAY
Of course Laetrile, or Vitamin B17, is not approved by the FDA, but not because it isn't beneficial – it is, as the information contained in this book demonstrates. No, Vitamin B17 has not been approved by the FDA simply because the FDA has been leaned on. That's the way it goes in the self-preserving, self-serving, conventional cancer business.

To put it bluntly, biddable FDA officials are only a phone call and a golfing lunch away from the NCI and the NIH. A classic example of these conflicts of interests and double standards can be appreciated when one learns that sodium fluoride is also not approved by the FDA due to its toxicity, and yet drug giant Proctor and Gamble and others can market the stuff in their toothpastes, claiming a pharmacological benefit, with complete impunity.

The UPHS statement on Laetrile is a fabrication. Such is the wealth of evidence overturning the conventional stance on Laetrile and Vitamin C, that one can only assume the UPHS statement falls into the following category:

---

[254] http://cancer.med.upenn.edu/pdq_html/6/engl/600093.html

FALSE SCIENTIFIC RESEARCH 'ENDANGERING THE PUBLIC' - *Independent News, 13th December 2000 - Doctors are fabricating research results to win grants and advance their careers, but the medical establishment is failing to protect the public from the menace of these scientific frauds, a committee of medical editors said yesterday. Eighty cases of fraudulent research have been detected in the past four years, and 30 have been investigated in the past year. In some cases, institutions have covered up wrongdoing to protect reputations....*

THE NUB OF IT

In an effort to subvert this mass-awakening to the horrors of conventional cancer treatments, a devious attack on all genuinely beneficial, natural (and therefore unpatentable) anti-cancer products is now being waged by a rather worried conventional cancer establishment. The ever-so-gentle slur on our most vital of vitamins, Vitamin C, will soon be extended to a wide range of essential minerals and vitamins.

This is just the beginning of the subtle, but concerted attack. The latest conventional legislation surrounding the codifying and banning of efficacious natural treatments is being instituted, purely because there is no money in these natural treatments for Big Pharma. It is profit before human health, but couched in respectable-looking, 'sciency' reports. And this veneer of respectability is fooling the unsuspecting minions lower down the UPHS research chain.

NAÏVE

The two UPHS officials Credence spoke to regarding Dr Blair's Vitamin C report were extremely pleasant, open and helpful and displayed no intention to supply misleading information. But both persons were entirely locked into their superiors' way of thinking. Media Relations officer Olivia Fermano was curious as to our interest into who funded the Vitamin C report. When we pointed out that if Dr Blair's funding could be traced to a pharmaceutical company producing conventional cancer treatments, then the results would have to be very seriously questioned, Ms Fermano was genuinely supportive. *"My goodness! That is a good question. I will be right back to you."*

Her word-for-word courteous reply, some two minutes later, was as follows: *"You had me genuinely worried for a few minutes there, Sir. But I am pleased to tell you that our funding came directly from the National Institutes for Health itself. I am so relieved."*

Ho Hum.

Similarly, Dr Garret Fitzgerald, chair of UPHS Centre for Cancer Pharmacy Department, stated: *"The evidence supporting Vitamin C as a useful adjunct in cancer treatment ranges from scant to non-existent. Linus Pauling's work was framed around a tenuous hypothesis only."*

Whilst the courtesy displayed by Ms Fermano and Dr Fitzgerald is commendable, their naivety is surely the result of them both working in a commercially cocooned workplace, purposefully insulated from the many success stories attributed to non-toxic, metabolic cancer treatments, and from the amazing health benefits accrued from consuming Vitamin C. For an excellent essay on this subject, please visit http://www.vitamincfoundation.org/mega_1_1.html and read an article entitled 'How Much Vitamin C Is Enough?'

For a more in-depth study of the conventional cancer industry, of the very good news concerning non-toxic, proven cancer treatments and of the benefits that Vitamin C, readers are encouraged to visit www.credence.org and take the cancer tour.

OTHER BOOK TITLES BY CREDENCE

Scared Sick of Cancer? Don't Be.
Get the Facts... and then get
on with your life !

CANCER: WHY WE'RE STILL DYING TO KNOW THE TRUTH
by Phillip Day

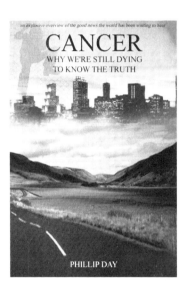

For more information on the truth behind cancer and Metabolic Therapy, our world-famous book, *Cancer: Why We're Still Dying to Know the Truth* is the excellent starting point. This overview title exposes the ongoing establishment cover-up over the failure of traditional cancer treatments and explains Metabolic Therapy (Vitamins B17/A&E/enzymes), the controversial treatment for cancer and its prevention. This book further details the amazing track record of nutrition and its role within the simple, combined protocol of Metabolic Therapy. Whether you have cancer, or are exercising prevention for you and your family, PLEASE get educated on this vital issue today.

Title: *Cancer: Why We're Still Dying to Know the Truth*
by Phillip Day
ISBN 0-9535012-4-8
First published in April 1999 by Credence Publications
Available at www.credence.org

B17 METABOLIC THERAPY IN THE PREVENTION AND CONTROL OF CANCER
- a technical manual -
compiled by Phillip Day

B17 METABOLIC THERAPY

in the prevention and
control of CANCER

a technical manual

compiled by
PHILLIP DAY

From the desks of some of the world's leading cancer scientists comes the empirical proof of Vitamin B17 and its co-factors in the treatment and prevention of cancer. These explosive findings have been the cause of the real cancer war, where vested interests have moved to vilify and denigrate nutrition in order to protect their highly lucrative cancer incomes.

- Find out why 18 'primitive' cultures do not get cancer in their isolated state.
- What three nutritional components have been found vital in the prevention and the treatment of cancer?
- What can you do to change your diet in ways which will give you maximum protection from cancer and other associated ailments?
- Why do animals not get cancer in the wild, yet succumb to it when 'domesticated' by humans?
- Discover the amazing research of Professor John Beard of Edinburgh University and American Biochemist Ernst T Krebs Jr which shows what cancer actually is. Remove your fear of this disease forever.
- Why are huge budgets continually spent on 'fighting the war against cancer' when this information has been in the public domain for 50 years?
- Examine the actual technical theses and trials carried out by doctors and scientists that validate this amazingly simple protocol.

- Find out what you can do today to join the global movement to eradicate cancer from the 21st century!

Phillip Day: *"Now comes the empirical information for doctors, scientists and laymen alike, which can be used at a local, state or global level to eradicate cancer and its heartache from the human race forever. Each of us has a chance today to be great – to remove far from us the greed, entrenched error and ignorance that has allowed cancer to flourish like an evil bloom in our midst. In a sense, cancer will remain around only as long as it takes humankind to achieve that rare level of maturity, when he will treasure his own well-being and that of his friends and loved ones before the tempting lure of wealth, prestige and renown."*

HEALTH WARS

by Phillip Day

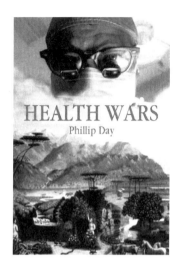

PRESS RELEASE: Western healthcare is now the third leading cause of death in Britain, according to a UK health research organisation. England-based Credence Research, citing statistics which demonstrate that drug-dominated medicine is now the third leading killer in most industrial nations, warns that the true death toll may be far higher than even its reported figures.

Credence Chief Executive Phillip Day states: *"225,000 Americans are killed every year by Western healthcare, according to the American Medical Association. In Britain, the official figure of 40,000 is in reality far higher, if you examine the proper markers. 1 in 5 Australians will be killed every year by their doctors, through incorrect drug-prescribing, botched medical procedures, infections in hospitals and, the main killer, <u>correct</u> drug prescribing. This worldwide allopathic catastrophe is well known to the authorities who, in reality, are unable to do much about it within the current healthcare system, for the reasons we report."*

Credence, whose recently released publication, *Health Wars*, deals with this unsettling phenomenon, states: *"90-95% of the diseases currently killing populations, at least in the industrial nations, are nutritional deficiency and/or toxin related conditions, such as heart disease, cancer, diabetes and stroke. To understand completely why medicine continues to fail with these problems, and worse, be guilty of its own unique slaughter of the citizenry, one need look no further than the fact that doctors receive almost no formal training in nutrition. Thus, doctors are not trained to understand the underlying metabolic problems of at least 90% of diseases, which can be treated effectively, even in their late stages, or completely prevented, using simple, and unfortunately un-patentable nutrition."*

On the toxin disease front, the medical establishment is equally dismissive and trivialises the real chemical and environmental causes, according to Credence. To illustrate why this happens, Day points out that the very industry responsible for producing and selling chemicals, which routinely kill and maim the public, also manufactures the public's medicines. *"Don't expect the chemical industry to gain a morality on this issue overnight. It is hamstrung by stark conflicts of interest. The urgent call for reform needed to prevent further tragedy on the scale we face must come from the public itself."*

On Credence's recently released book, Day declares: *"The purpose of 'Health Wars' is to highlight these problems and to urge citizens to pressure their governments for immediate reform. Compounding its failures, British healthcare has ironically been brought to its knees by the crippling costs of the very drugs and treatments, which have been, and continue to be, the main instigators of these frightening death statistics. Credence has been looking at mortality. But how many citizens out there have been crippled or maimed by healthcare practices, such as vaccinations, errant drug prescribing and unnecessary surgeries? Recent reports show that the NHS must budget every year for at least £2.8 billion in compensation claims alone. That's enough to build and fully staff 28 new hospitals every twelve months."*

Credence states that medical science has known for years that the answers to heart disease, cancer, stroke and other illnesses lie completely in nutrition and lifestyle changes, not radical surgeries, toxic drugs or radiation. To prove this point, the company cites at least 18 cultures alive today who do not apparently suffer from these health problems. *"Interestingly,"* Day elaborates, *"we tend to call these peoples 'primitive' and 'less developed'. But they know enough about nutrition to ensure that they survive in sterling health, in many cases to over 100 years of age. The authorities know this too, and do nothing. Why? Because Western healthcare today is a multi-trillion-dollar industry worldwide, and you cannot pay CEO salaries and shareholder dividends using apples, oranges and chemical-free, organic vegetation."*

Day believes that health reform is inevitable, and that the public can do much to precipitate the process by getting educated and politically active: *"A proper healthcare industry must have nutritional education at its heart,"* he states. *"This is the most basic body science. We are what we eat. But the people will have to fight a war with their industrial and political peers first, in order to secure the return of their unalienable right to drink fresh, uncontaminated water, to eat fresh, uncontaminated food and to breathe fresh, uncontaminated air."*

Title: *Health Wars*
by Phillip Day
ISBN 1-904015-01-8 (325 pages)
First edition published June 2001 by Credence Publications
Available at www.credence.org

FOOD FOR THOUGHT

compiled by Phillip Day

Need a guide on where to go with your food? What better way to embrace the dietary concepts laid down in *Cancer:Why We're Still Dying to Know the Truth* and *Health Wars* than to obtain a copy of our official recipe book.

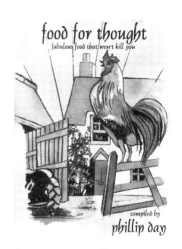

This delightful guide takes you through the main concepts of acid/alkali, Vitamin B17 dishes, the proper combining of foods, the problems with meat and dairy in excessive amounts, fruit consumption techniques, a host of detox menus, 5-10% meat and dairy recipes, snacks, pro-active sickness dieting, children's dishes and proper supplementation. Whether you are suffering or just want to make a change for your extended future, sensible nutrition comes to life in *Food For Thought*, bringing you the most delicious foods that WON'T KILL YOU!

Title: *Food for Thought*
Compiled by Phillip Day
ISBN 1-904015-04-2
First published in August 2001 by Credence Publications
Available at www.credence.org

PLAGUE, PESTILENCE AND THE PURSUIT OF POWER

by Steven Ransom

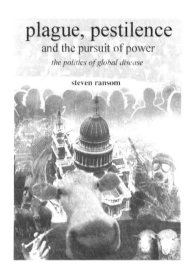

Almost every day, it seems, we are hearing reports of some 'highly infectious' disease breaking out somewhere across the world - the recent flu pandemics, AIDS decimating Africa, tuberculosis on the rise again, measles, and meningitis on the increase. And in the animal kingdom, we've seen Bovine Spongiform Encephalopathy (BSE), poultry flu, swine fever, more BSE and now foot and mouth, wreaking havoc across our countryside. One could be forgiven for thinking that we are quite literally surrounded by virulent illness. But not everything is as it seems – not by a long way.

In this book, we discover that these so-called 'epidemics' are NOT the deadly illnesses we have been led to believe by our respective governments, national papers and news programs. With all the above-mentioned illnesses, the facts being disseminated have been grossly misleading, accompanied, in many instances, by a deliberate intent to scare and deceive. Welcome to the shocking world of the politically manufactured epidemic - the 'psycho-plague'.

The formula is quite simple. Using the mainstream media as their chosen vehicle for change, powerful vested interests are deliberately instigating national and international fearsome headlines. Through these channels, the problem – the epidemic – the psycho-plague, is manufactured. A crisis has now been firmly embedded into the mind of the populace. **"We must have a solution!"** we cry. Lo and behold, a governmental/corporate solution is speedily proffered.

In reality, the epidemic needing 'swift state intervention' has been nothing more than a Trojan Horse either for creating immense profit for various pharmaceutical industries or, as we shall discover, for ushering in unsavoury, global super-state ideology. Throughout this whole process, we are being taught what to think about health and disease, but not how.

In examining the facts laid out before us, we soon realise that our battle is not so much against pathological disease, as against corrupt and self-serving desires, birthed in the minds of man. This book contains the supporting evidence to make this case. You are invited to consider the evidence for yourself.

But this book also maps out a positive way forward. For, in discovering the true nature and causes of these 'epidemics', a longer lasting remedy can now be planned for the future.

Plague, Pestilence and the Pursuit of Power is dedicated to those who want to find out what really goes on behind the closed doors of Big Business and Big Government and to those who wish to see truth reign in conventional science and medicine.

Title: *Plague, Pestilence and the Pursuit of Power*
by Steven Ransom
ISBN 0-9535012-8-0 (205 pages)
First published in June 2001 by Credence Publications
Available at www.credence.org

All titles can also be obtained from the distributor whose details are in the *Contacts!* section of this book.

WORLD WITHOUT AIDS
by Steven Ransom & Phillip Day

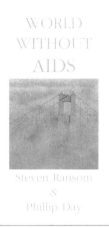

One of the greatest scandals in medicine today surrounds the classification of AIDS as an infectious disease. The supposed pathogen, human immunodeficiency virus (HIV), despite much fanfare and fear-mongering, has never been isolated according to any recognised and appropriate scientific procedure. And so, from a scientific standpoint, HIV can be deemed not to exist. Since Dr Robert Gallo's so-called 'discovery of HIV' in 1984 (at which he displayed a fake 'image' for which he was later convicted of science fraud), no empirical proof for the existence of HIV has ever been furnished to the scientific establishment. Monetary rewards for 'The Missing Virus' remain uncollected by the conventional scientific community for a properly isolated HI virus, according to all the normal rules.

All the evidence shows that immune suppression ('AIDS') in the Western World is primarily brought on by long-term recreational or pharmaceutical drug toxicity **AND IS NOT INFECTIOUS OR SEXUALLY TRANSMITTED**. So-called Third World or 'African' 'AIDS' is nothing more than the cynical reclassification of diseases that have always killed Africans, namely: dysentery, cholera, malnutrition, TB, malaria, typhoid and parasitic infections, brought on by the frequently contaminated water supplies which Africans and inhabitants of other nations are forced to tolerate. To add to this injustice, Africans are almost always classified as 'AIDS carriers' by the authorities through visual diagnosis only. This arbitrary, World Health Organisation-approved method of diagnosis is known as the Bangui method.

In order to be deemed an AIDS carrier under Bangui, one need only be suffering from diarrhoea, fever and demonstrate a 10% weight loss over a two-month period. These symptoms can of course relate to almost all of the above-mentioned diseases that were (and still are) common across Africa prior to all the dramatic AIDS headlines. Illnesses that are relatively simple to treat have now been cynically clustered under the AIDS umbrella. The collective impact of this manoeuvre serves only to reinforce the errant belief that HIV is decimating Africa and other poorer nations. It also gives more credibility to the growing number of reports that AIDS is re-emerging in the West.

In the West, AIDS is hardly less scandalous. Many unwitting victims are drawn into the AIDS nightmare by inadvertently triggering a 'positive' on one of two main tests given to patients today. The ELISA (Enzyme-Linked Immuno-Absorbent Assay) and Western Blot tests are designed to highlight the presence of the supposed HIV, not by identifying the virus itself, but by indicating the presence of antibodies in the blood allegedly unique to, and stimulated by the virus. But as we have already discovered, all the diagnostic methods employed by the recognised laboratories are far from specific. Prominent AIDS researcher Christine Maggiore, herself a victim of these fraudulent tests, states the major problem as follows:

"Both tests are non-specific to HIV antibodies and are highly inaccurate. Non-specific means that these tests respond to a great number of non-HIV antibodies, microbes, bacteria and other conditions that are often found in the blood of normal, healthy people. A reaction to any one of these other antibodies and conditions will result in an HIV positive diagnosis. A simple illness like a cold or the flu can cause a positive reading on an HIV test. A flu shot or other vaccine can also create positive results. Having or having had herpes or hepatitis may produce a positive test, as can a vaccination for hepatitis B. Exposure to diseases such as tuberculosis and malaria commonly cause false positive results, as do the presence of tape worms and other parasites. Conditions such as alcoholism, liver disease and blood that is highly oxidated through drug use may be interpreted as the presence of HIV antibodies. Pregnancy and prior pregnancy can also cause a positive result." [255]

---

[255] Maggiore, Christine, *What if Everything You Thought You Knew About AIDS Was Wrong?* Alive and Well, Studio City, CA 90604, USA

The triggering of an HIV positive will lead invariably to prescriptions for the deadly cell toxins AZT, ddI and other 'HIV' drugs, which have an appalling history of causing the very immune deficiencies they were supposedly designed to prevent. South African barrister Anthony Brink remarks:

"In truth, AZT makes you feel like you're dying. That's because on AZT you are. How can a deadly cell toxin conceivably make you feel better as it finishes you, by stopping your cells from dividing, by ending this vital process that distinguishes living things from dead things? Not for nothing does AZT come with a skull and cross-bones label when packaged for laboratory use."[256]

And indeed that is the case. With a skull and cross-bones on the outer label and a reminder to wear suitable protective clothing when handling, the inner contents of the AZT packaging include the following side-effects advisory notice:

WHOLE BODY: abdominal pain, back pain, body odour, chest pain, chills, edema of the lip, fever, flu symptoms, hyperalgesia.
CARDIOVASCULAR: syncope, vasodilation.
GASTROINTESTINAL: bleeding gums, constipation, diarrhoea, dysphagia, edema of the tongue, eructation, flatulence, mouth ulcer, rectal haemorrhage.
HAEMIC AND LYMPHATIC: lymphadenopathy.
MUSCULOSKELETAL: arthralgia, muscle spasm, tremor, twitch.
NERVOUS: anxiety, confusion, depression, dizziness, emotional lability, loss of mental acuity, nervousness, paresthesia, somnolence, vertigo.
RESPIRATORY: cough, dyspnea, epistaxis, hoarseness, pharyngitis, rhinitis, sinusitis.
SKIN: rash, sweat, urticaria.
SPECIAL SENSES: amblyopia, hearing loss, photophobia, taste perversion.
UROGENITAL: dysuria, polyuria, urinary frequency, urinary hesitancy.

---

[256] Brink, Anthony, *AZT and Heavenly Remedies*, Rethinking AIDS Homepage: www.rethinkingaids.com

Phillip Day spent eight years in Los Angeles and San Francisco working with those deemed HIV positive by the medical establishment. In all cases, he reports, their plight could be laid at the door of excessive lifestyles, recreational or pharmaceutical drug terrorism and a general lack of education surrounding the true nature and causes of immune deficiency. Their sure and ready remedy was to move towards wellness with a properly constructed regimen of sound nutrition and supplementation. The full Credence report is contained in *World Without AIDS*, the result of 15 years' research into this tragically misunderstood realm of medical fraud, injustice and error.

It seems though that with these profitable AIDS treatments, the fraud, injustice and error is set to continue. A mandatory AIDS vaccine is looming.

***REPORT PREDICTS MASSIVE RESISTANCE TO MANDATORY AIDS VACCINE** - Wes Vernon, NewsMax, 24th June, 2001 - A new report predicts massive resistance to a mandatory AIDS vaccine that is coming to the US in the next few years. Millions of parents would refuse to have their children vaccinated by any variation of an HIV/AIDS shot, the Committee to Protect Medical Freedom said at a news conference Wednesday. Jim Turner, a Washington attorney and expert on the swine flu vaccine scandal of the 1970s, lent his support, as did Barbara Lee Fisher, co-founder and president of the National Vaccine Information Center. The thrust of the report, written by Clifford Kincaid, is that there's big money in rushing an AIDS vaccine to market, some of it tied up in conflict-of-interest questions involving the promoters and their connections with companies that stand to benefit.*

Barbara Loe Fisher, co-founder of the National Vaccine Information Center, reports that a member of the federal committee that recommends vaccines for children had said that an AIDS vaccine would be tested and then forced on all 12-year-old children. Neal Halsey, M.D., chairman of the American Academy of Pediatrics (AAP) Committee on Infectious Diseases, reminded HIV vaccine researchers and developers at a meeting in February 1997 of an advisory committee of the federal Centers for Disease Control that CDC plans to target 11- to 12-year-old children for "universal application" of an HIV vaccine.

The Kincaid study says, "...babies are being used as guinea pigs now." The National Institute for Allergy and Infectious Diseases, under the auspices of the federal Department of Health and Human Services, is sponsoring an HIV vaccine test on babies born to HIV-infected women." [257]

If this wasn't bad enough, every expectant mothers in the UK is now being recommended to take an 'HIV' test. In some states in the US, the test is mandatory. Submitting to this test will result in these women standing a chance of being deemed HIV positive, simply because of the mother's heightened levels of antibody activity picked up by these tests. The resultant medication is as catastrophic to the baby as it is to the mother. For this reason, Credence has issued the following advisory leaflet for the urgent attention of all expectant mothers and all those planning to start a family. The leaflet is available in printer-friendly format at www.credence.org

* * * * *

HEALTH WARNING TO EXPECTANT MOTHERS

If you have recently become pregnant, you will be recommended to take an HIV test as part of a standardised ante-natal care package.[258] This test is highly inaccurate and remains scientifically unproven. It should be refused on the following grounds.

1) All manufacturers of these tests include the following or similar disclaimer with their test kits: "At present, there is no recognised standard for establishing the presence or absence of antibodies to HIV-1 and HIV- 2 in human blood."[259]

---

[257] The full report can be found at:
http://www.newsmax.com/archives/articles/2001/6/20/152903.shtml
[258] Refer to "Review of antenatal testing services", NHS Regional Office, London, UK Dept of Health. Recommending the HIV test became UK national policy in July 1999, and is now mandatory in some US states.
[259] The above disclaimer is included in all Abbott 'AXSYM' Aids tests at the time of writing, the world's leading supplier of AIDS test kits.

2) The reason for this disclaimer is because the AIDS test does not measure the presence of a virus.[260] The AIDS test has been designed to detect levels of antibody activity in the blood. Antibody activity in the blood stream is a normal occurrence in humans, but is being misinterpreted by the AIDS test as indicative of the presence of HIV.

3) As a result of this misinterpretation, healthy individuals are being wrongly diagnosed as HIV positive. Since this information has come to light, in excess of 60 different medical conditions have been recorded that can give rise to a false HIV positive reading. These separate conditions include flu, flu vaccination, malaria, tetanus vaccination, Hepatitis A and B, Hepatitis vaccinations, alcohol and drug use, recent viral infections and even pregnancy.[261] Receiving a spurious but emotionally devastating diagnosis of HIV positive will prompt your doctor to recommend a course of anti-HIV drugs. Known as protease inhibitors or anti-retrovirals, these drugs are highly toxic. They have the well-documented capacity to harm the mother, and also severely to deform and even kill the unborn child. [262]

The current level of spending on AIDS drugs in the Western World is phenomenal. So too are the profits enjoyed by the AIDS drug manufacturers. As a result, the information contained in this advisory leaflet is largely being ignored by the medical establishment. Sadly, this is not an unexpected reaction. The pursuit of profit at the expense of health, the wilful employment of flawed medical procedures, the administration of dangerously toxic drugs to expectant mothers, the disregard for the plight of thousands upon thousands of wrongly diagnosed people, and a refusal by the medical establishment to listen to sound contrary evidence or to admit medical negligence - all these

---

[260] Monetary rewards offered to leading organisations within the scientific community by concerned organisations for reasonable evidence that HIV exists remain uncollected.

[261] Johnson, Christine, *Continuum Magazine*, September 1996. Maggiore, Christine, *What if Everything You Knew about AIDS was Wrong?* An Alive and Well Publication, April 2000. Ransom & Day, *World Without AIDS*, Credence Publications, July 2000.

[262] Kumar et al, *Journal of Acquired Immune Deficiency Syndromes*, 7; 1034-9, 1994. *JAMA Journal of American Medical Association*, Jan 5th 2000, Incidence of liver damage. *World Without AIDS*. AZT and enlarged craniums in infants. Refer to www.virusmyth.com for a more comprehensive list of scientific references which catalogue the damage caused by AIDS drugs.

are the hallmarks of that once-respected drug, thalidomide. Do not allow either yourself or your child to face the possibility of becoming another heartbreaking medical statistic.

WORLD WITHOUT AIDS

World Without AIDS dismantles one of the world's greatest fears and lays bare the deceit, fraudulent science and needless fearmongering that lie at the heart of this supposed global epidemic. Over ten years in the making, this impeccably researched book gives an eye-opening account of what vested interests can get away with, given a trusting public, an almost limitless supply of money and scant scruples. It also explains the non-existence of HIV, the bankruptcy of the HIV test, the real causes of immune suppression, the AIDS-devastating-Africa myth and the appalling dangers of the establishment-approved medications prescribed to those who have been written off as 'HIV positive'.

Title: *World Without AIDS*
by Steve Ransom and Phillip Day
ISBN 0-9535012-5-6
First published in June 2000 by Credence Publications
Available through credence.org

CAMPAIGN FOR TRUTH IN MEDICINE
"a force for change"

WHAT IS CTM?

Campaign for Truth in Medicine is a worldwide organisation dedicated to pressing for change in areas of science and medicine where entrenched scientific error, ignorance or vested interests are costing lives. Its ranks comprise doctors, scientists, researchers, biochemists, politicians, industry executives and countless members of the world public, all of whom have made one

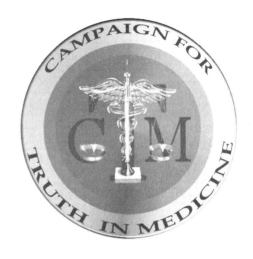

observation in common. They have recognised that, in certain key areas of global disease, drug treatments and overall healthcare philosophy, the medical, chemical and political establishments are pursuing the wrong course with the maximum of precision, even when their own legitimate and crudite scientific research has illustrated the dangers of pursuing these courses.

CTM BACKS ITS PEOPLE'S CHARTER

CTM's People's Charter catalogues these key problem areas - for example AIDS, cancer, heart disease and vaccinations - where the preponderance of evidence demonstrates severe cause for concern over deadly errors in basic science, resulting in needless loss of life. CTM's charter also highlights industry's every-day use of potentially harmful contaminants and biohazards, such as toothpaste's sodium fluoride, shampoo's sodium lauryl sulphate and cosmetic's propylene glycol, which have long been linked to long-term serious health risks and death. CTM's purpose is to present this damning evidence to its members, to the public at large and to the establishments and individuals involved in these errors, in order to press for immediate change and cessation of their use for the benefit of humanity. The

People's Charter is periodically amended to reflect current issues and new areas of concern.

CTM STANDS FOR TRUTH
For decades members of the public and a significant proportion of their medical and scientific professionals have become increasingly angry and frustrated at what they see as establishment indifference and even downright hostility towards much-needed changes in healthcare, especially in areas where the proven solution is substantially less profitable than the current status quo.

PROMOTING THE TRUTH
CTM believes in promoting the truth in these matters, thereby exposing those morally bankrupt and compromised politicians, corporations and individuals responsible. This method of action is viewed as a top priority. CTM is dedicated to pushing for immediate change, in order that immediate relief from many of the diseases and their causes, currently afflicting us, may be implemented, the remedies for which, in certain cases, have been a matter of existing scientific knowledge for decades.

The Journal of the American Medical Association (JAMA) implicitly reports that western healthcare, along with its drugs, treatments and hospitals, is now the third leading cause of death in the United States, next to heart disease and cancer. If we examine this astonishing fact, also highlighted by US consumer advocate Ralph Nader in the early 1990's, we come to realise that the Western healthcare paradigm is adopted by almost all developed nations and many other developing countries around the world. Thus this tragic statistic of iatrogenic death can be fairly considered to be global in application.

This would be serious enough on its own, yet the true extent of this orthodox medical catastrophe is unfortunately far more devastating. Western medical establishments are in possession of key life-saving information that can immediately and drastically reduce current and future global incidences of cancer, heart disease, AIDS and other treatable, non-fatal conditions. But in almost all cases these institutions have chosen neither to adopt these measures, train their healthcare practitioners in these practices, nor publicize the latter to a generally trusting world populace. Thus these government personnel and their associated medical luminaries, who have wilfully kept this life-saving information from their doctors and the public, may justifiably be exposed for becoming the leading cause of death across the planet today.

CTM STANDS FOR DIRECT ACTION
CTM believes that, in certain cases, legitimate direct action is warranted against these institutions and individuals to halt their wilful and harmful actions and hold them to account. In these circumstances, CTM calls upon its membership to organise and act in a unified, lawful and mature fashion to bring these matters to the attention of the mass communications media, government leaders and heads of state through demonstrations and other appropriate action. CTM is dedicated to being part of the people's movement in this regard; a powerful and irresistible force for change, compelling vital reform TODAY for a safer and healthier world for our children and children's children.

CTM IS FREE FROM VESTED INTEREST FUNDING
Through its network of worldwide professional contacts, CTM has constant access to well-researched information on key health issues. CTM brings its members highly readable and jargon-free information, such as that contained in this book.

CTM HAS ALL THE NECESSARY CONTACTS
...at local and central government/corporate level, responsible for particular health legislation and legislative change. Names, addresses, contact details and relevant template letters are supplied with all CTM newsletters.

CTM IS A HEALTH ADVOCACY ORGANISATION
with purpose and direction. It is a conduit through which the individual minority voice can become a powerful and respected, collective majority voice for change.

WHAT YOU CAN DO NOW

CTM invites you to visit its web-site to learn more about how you can join this worldwide movement FOR FREE and receive regular bulletins and further information on these fascinating subjects as they develop. Be part of a different future. One that celebrates life!

**Campaign for Truth in Medicine
PO Box 3
Tonbridge,
Kent,
TN 12 9ZY UK
e-mail: info@campaignfortruth.com
www.campaignfortruth.com**

CONTACTS! CONTACTS! CONTACTS!

Readers wishing to make inquiries into purchasing more copies of this book can use the contact details below:

> US Auto Orders: (309) 416 8714
> UK Orders: (01622) 832386
> Int'l Orders: +44 1622 832386
> UK Fax: (01622) 833314
> www.credence.org
> e-mail: sales@credence.org

HEALTH REVIEW AND FREE INFORMATION PACK
What other book entitles you to a free magazine subscription and regular e-mail updates completely free? If you have not received these and have purchased this book, contact us on the above numbers.

Credence also sends hundreds of free information packs throughout the world every month to those who have requested them either for themselves or for interested friends and relatives. Those who receive such packs will receive our seasonal magazine Health Review, informing the reader of the latest developments on this and other interesting health topics. If you would like to take advantage of this service, please supply the relevant mailing address details to our head office address below:

Credence Publications
PO Box 3
TONBRIDGE
Kent TN12 9ZY
England
infopack@credence.org

ECLUB BULLETINS

Twice each month, the Campaign for Truth in Medicine sends out the EClub Internet bulletin to thousands of subscribers worldwide. This highly informative e-mail newsletter is available FREE to customers who have purchased this book or who have requested EClub. This online bulletin contains the latest news and research on cancer and other vital health topics. DO NOT BE WITHOUT THIS GREAT RESOURCE! If you wish to subscribe, log on to the Campaign site at www.campaignfortruth.com and click the 'Join CTM' tab to complete your free application.

INDEX

W